D1519285

Activities
and
Action
in
Groupwork

The *Social Work with Groups* series

Series Editors: Catherine P. Papell and Beulah Rothman

Activities
and
Action
in
Groupwork

Ruth Middleman
Guest Editor

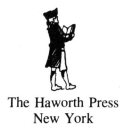

The Haworth Press
New York

Activities and Action in Groupwork has also been published as *Social Work with Groups*, Volume 6, Number 1, Spring 1983.

The Haworth Press, Inc., 28 East 22 Street, New York, NY 10010

Library of Congress Cataloging in Publication Data
Main entry under title:

Activities and action in groupwork.

   (Social work with groups; v. 6, no. 1)
   Bibliography: p.
   Includes index.
   1. Social group work—Addresses, essays, lectures. 2. Social action—Addresses, essays, lectures. I. Middleman, Ruth R. II. Series: Social work with groups (Haworth Press); v. 6, no. 1.
HV45.S63   vol. 6, no. 1 [HV45]   361.4s   83-309
ISBN 0-86656-228-1   [361.4]

Activities and Action in Groupwork

Social Work with Groups
Volume 6, Number 1

CONTENTS

BOOK REVIEWS

HENRY W. MAIER, PhD, *School of Social Work, University of Washington, Seattle*
RUTH R. MIDDLEMAN, EdD, *Raymond A. Kent School of Social Work, University of Louisville, Kentucky*
HELEN NORTHEN, PhD, *School of Social Work, University of Southern California, Los Angeles*
RUBY B. PERNELL, DSW, *School of Applied Social Sciences, Case Western Reserve University, Cleveland*
HELEN PHILLIPS, DSW, *School of Social Work, University of Pennsylvania, Philadelphia*
HERMAN RESNICK, PhD, *School of Social Work, University of Washington, Seattle*
SHELDON ROSE, PhD, *School of Social Work, University of Wisconsin, Madison*
JANICE H. SCHOPLER, MSW, *School of Social Work, University of North Carolina, Chapel Hill*
LAWRENCE SHULMAN, EdD, *School of Social Work, University of British Columbia, Vancouver, Canada*
MARY LOUISE SOMERS, DSW, *School of Social Service Administration, University of Chicago*
EMANUEL TROPP, MSSW, *School of Social Work, Virginia Commonwealth University, Richmond*
ROBERT VINTER, PhD, *School of Social Work, University of Michigan, Ann Arbor*
CELIA B. WEISMAN, DSW, *Wurzweiler School of Social Work, Yeshiva University New York*
GERTRUDE WILSON, MA, *University of California, Berkeley*

Activities
and
Action
in
Groupwork

Editorial

This special issue, "Activities and Action in Groupwork," is an exemplar of the long-standing devotion of group workers to the idea of the inseparability of content and process. For the group worker and the members, translating this idea into actual practice requires creative effort.

Doing together is the essential substance of human interaction. *What people do together* constitutes the inventiveness of human social experience and the primary stuff for forming perceptions of self and others. This issue deals with this creative effort in the social group work process.

That Ruth Middleman is the editor of this special issue is indisputably appropriate. For group workers, she is a principal contemporary theoretician, conceptualizing for us the creative dynamics in programming. For the social work profession as a whole, through her writings and her experiential demonstrations and teaching, she has kept alive the group work conviction about activity and has enhanced it through broader application and more highly developed theory.

The writings in this special issue illustrate three essential principles in relation to the use of activity in group work practice:

1. Activities are approached with a view to their versatility, and adaptability, subject to change, modification, or development through spontaneous as well as planned processes.
2. Activities are viewed with regard to their attributes for meeting individual and group needs in the spirit of enhancing mutuality rather than competition.
3. Activities result from responsiveness to the emerging resources in the group and the situations and are valued for their symbolic representation of the life of the specific group.

Social Work with Groups is honored to present this special issue to its readers.

CPP
BR

1

Guest Editorial

You may wonder why there should be a special issue devoted to this component of group work. Several of the articles here could have "made it" on their own merits in a regular issue of *Social Work with Groups*. And yet, the announced call for papers on the theme of action/activities probably encouraged some of our contributors to write and submit what they were doing with more hope that their article would "see the light of day." For, despite the *experiential explosion* of the past 20 years and despite the widespread public awareness of the right side of the brain—of the importance of the intuitive, the non-rational, the spontaneous, the creative, and the expression of these personal attributes, there is still a reluctance to examine program *qua* program in the literature.

The record of the work devoted to pursuing the nitty-gritty, the ordinary activities of every day living, and the painstaking involvement and patience demanded of the group worker to engage with the group participants on their own terms and turf remain a shadowy side of group work. Hopefully, by beaming a spot light on *what groups do,* we shall see what is "old" and what is "new" in the use of program with groups. There is an irony here. The encouragement of a focus on activities was a reach-out of sorts to solicit a special kind of group work. This reach-out brought a deepened view of reach-out! That is, you will see here an unusual amount of work with the hard-to-reach, with populations where mistrust and inaccessibility to ordinary helpers prevailed, with populations aptly described by Casey and Cantor as ones that "make the community uncomfortable." In one way or another we will be seeing persons whose need and pain are great and who are not pushing in the doors of offices nor paying to be helped.

Let me start with this little thought:

I remember and I was.
I feel and I am
I do and I become.[1]

---

[1]Joan M. Erikson, *Activity Recovery, Growth.* New York: Norton, 1976, p. 250. This book is recommended to all who want to read more about the use of activities.

The emphasis in these articles is on what groups of people *do* and what such doing may help them become. You will note as one common theme that the activities led to discussion—a point specially highlighted by Delgado in relation to Hispanics, by Darrow and Lynch in relation to picture taking with early teens, and by Casey and Cantor with their "big kids." This is an "old" theme seen afresh in its vitality to connect members and worker(s) in pursuit of group and individual goals and with such issues as control, authority, and planning. The bowling alley, skit, camera, bus ride, auto cruise, trip, or celebration are, in this scenario, mere handles to grasp and hold onto "for dear life" as group and worker(s) together venture from these events to discussions and explorations through which their development and movement will be known.

Some general observations are in order. The contributors represent a sweep of backgrounds: from BSW to PhD, from worker, specialist, planner/consultant, to professor. Two of the articles are described as "experiments." The articles are diverse so far as time frame is concerned: Katz's jazz performance was a one session affair while Casey and Cantor offer us a rare glimpse of what can happen to a group over a five year span, with boys who began at age 12 and ended when they were seventeen. Some of the discussions start with the activity (television production, poetry, photography, jam session) and move from its potentials to those involved with the activity. In other instances, it is the population first—the hard-to-reach, acting out adolescent, the underserved Hispanics, the pregnant teenager—and then there is a move to find ways to interest the persons through carefully constructed involvement with activities.

I was impressed by the seriousness of the problematic situations that these articles addressed. I noticed the preponderance of teenage work represented herein, with groups that were coping with the ordinary anguish of this life-phase as well as the many "special" issues that went along with their marginal situations. Teenagers have never been terribly eager to have adult influence. Several of the groups you will meet in this issue are mixed racially—white, black, Hispanic. It is exciting to see such sensitive, skilled group work still happening with these populations.

As you will see, activities for these groups are not fun and games, diversional, recreational, or escapist. Rather, they are hard work; they are lifeblood. For example, Getzel talks of old peoples' transmitting generational experience, creating contemporary epic poems which link past and future, handle loss, and help them redefine themselves at a richer, more complex level. Kilburn deals with life-saving information and the development of "family" networks for social support and crisis help which the young, single parent needs. The concreteness of the network expressed in the annual reunion picnic where 35–50 parents and up to 75 children gather, much like the family events, parties, and celebrations planned by the Hispanic groups, attest to the basic role of planned activities in the groups' lives.

The seriousness of the picture "taking" and "snapping" described by Darrow and Lynch is far from a trivial activity. We see here the move from the fearful, anxious beginning of young teens, afraid to take the camera out of the box, to the careless and random shooting, to the planned photography plus the talk about body image, racial, and sexual identities. Delgado describes in rich detail the "culturally sensitive activities" needed for successful work with Hispanics and offers an enormously useful typology of activities as well as an impressive conceptual scheme which interrelates the variables of group stages, activities, and cultural requirements.

The Israeli disadvantaged youth from problem-ridden backgrounds described in Shinar's article come to realize that the environment is not totally hostile to them and that they can be accepted by the "legitimate" environment. These insights were a by-product of their work in writing and producing television programs. Not only did they deal with the creative and technical components of their 10–15 minute programs, but they worked on "difficulties of self-awareness and image, problematic relationships, and the lack of certain functional values, attitudes, and skills." And in Casey and Cantor's group of delinquent and pre-delinquent boys, they may have started out thinking their group was for having fun and keeping out of trouble, but they ended up posting additional goals in their final self-evaluation: "some sort of counselling, facing a problem as a group, learning to get along with other people, and taking different roles!" It was, indeed, moving to read of their natural ambivalence at ending their group. Even though they knew it had served its purpose, they teased that they might revert to breaking and entering again so as to show their need for the group.

Perhaps these snips and bits suggest the richness and diversity in store for you in this volume. There is more. Kilburn presents an elaborate listing of the components of a outreach program for suspicious, pregnant teens (and their mothers!) that illustrates a breadth of planning considerations and contingencies that can easily be generalized to other hesitant populations. Katz's account of the jazz performance is included as a rare example of careful examination of the components and potentials of a communicative medium. She discusses three tasks which comprise a spontaneous performance of an ensemble of five virtual strangers. This is followed by a discussion concerned with decision making, cohesion, leadership, and other group dynamics, a written questionnaire plus some final reflection and analysis of this experience in relation to small group theory. The quest for further knowledge and meticulous study of small group interaction should serve as inspiration and incentive to others of us and renew our awareness that understanding the small group never ends. There is much to explore.

I want to call special attention to two other insights which these articles stimulated in me. For one, I noted how many of the articles offer some format of stages of group development as backdrop for viewing and understanding differences in activities, i.e., in accord with group movement over time. (And possibly the choice of activity is instrumental to this very group movement!) The connection between activities and group stages represents, I believe, an advance in theory building and development. The use of program activities within the intricate fabric of group life is more sophisticated than in the past. To this extent, these authors are contributing to theory-building. As another stunning piece of theory development, I applaud Casey and Cantor's formulation of their role in relation to activities, as the "protectors and keepers of the members' control." Their spontaneous use of the group's experience, their re-active leadership style in relation to the activities (they hold the group to making a choice so long as it is unanimous) is a break-through that merits study and replication attempts.

Getzel writes of the values of poetry creating in a way that is, itself, lyrical and passionate. He reminds us that the arts are also ends, have products and not merely means to some therapeutic ends. He implores that we view the product as an important achievement in its own right and gives us several products to appreciate, the poems of old persons which may "liberate the spiritual in this age of false spirits and disappointments." The point is well taken. The wonder of doing and producing and playing and laughing and eating and all the exciting, the exacting, the excruciating, the exasperating, the expansive things that groups do are part of what has made group work special.

The action and activities are learning, are becoming passports, are life. What groups *do* or produce link to the more sober requirements for valued participation in the world of affairs. The linkage to competence, to self-value, and to appreciation by others is well established. These achievements are the expression of consciousness. They are deliberate and purposeful, valuable in their energy/matter, as memories or as actualities.

Feldenkrais devoted a lifetime to exploring movement. He claims that movement most distinguishes animal life from vegetation. In the basic requirements of self-reproduction, self-maintenance, and self-preservation, animals are active while vegetables are passive. I was struck by this notion of the basic quality of activity. Is there a connection here to our thinking about group work? I leave this to you to ponder.

Ruth Middleman
Professor
Raymond A. Kent School of Social Work
Louisville, KY

Group Work
with Hard-to-Reach Adolescents:
The Use of Member Initiated
Program Selection

Richard D. Casey
Leon Cantor

ABSTRACT. Treatment of the adolescent population, especially delinquent and pre-delinquent youth, has been a difficult challenge in the mental health field. Traditional treatment modalities not suited to unmotivated, verbally unsophisticated teenagers have generally bypassed them. We describe here the adaptation of streetwork and therapeutic activity group practice to this population. Focus is on the flexible use of member initiated program selection as a dynamic group work tool.

Introduction

Working with hard-to-reach, acting-out adolescents has been one of the more difficult challenges in the field of social work. The modes of acting-out and the specific issues may vary from urban to suburban to rural settings, but all communities have angry, nonverbal, and unmotivated adolescents and pre-adolescents. Each community must find ways of dealing with this population.

There has been a good deal written about streetwork and about therapeutic activity groups. In the former the worker is seen as the link connecting alienated youth with opportunities that will make better functioning members of society (Bernstein, 1964, pp. 27-28). In the latter the leader is seen as the designer of activities appropriate to the needs and goals of a carefully structured group process (Middleman, 1980, pp. 141-145). This article is an effort to

Richard D. Casey, Group Work Coordinator, and Leon Cantor, Group Worker, are at the Arlington Youth Consultation Center, 12 Prescott St., Arlington, MA 02174.

bridge the gap between a streetwise population and theories of group planning. The model of group development used is one developed at Boston University School of Social Work (Garland et al., 1973, pp. 17-71). It described five stages: Pre-affiliation, Power and Control, Intimacy, Differentiation, and Separation.

Our agency has run many controlled in-house groups. It is also our mandate to work with those teens who make the community uncomfortable. These young people are not interested in coming to the clinic, so the workers must go to them. This means being available in terms of environment, behavior and attitudes, and is reflected in outreach into neighborhoods, schools, and homes. It does not mean adopting the youth's attitudes and behavior, but we emphasize awareness and acceptance of these differences. These youth are not interested in activities suggested by the workers, so the workers, within bounds, must use activities suggested by the youth. Yielding control in this area is a key to connecting and working with such groups. The challenge is to be spontaneous and creative with the available activities to make the experience work.

Development of Member Initiated Program

The group began partly in response to a referred boy's fear of treatment, and partly in response to a community need. Paul, age 12, was referred to the agency following a break-in at his elementary school in which several small animals were killed. He was ordered by his juvenile probation officer to meet weekly with the worker. Paul, however, was too anxious to make use of the meetings, even when we left the clinic for a more casual atmosphere. Meanwhile, the agency was becoming increasingly aware of acting-out behavior in the housing project community on the part of twelve and thirteen year old boys. An activity group seemed to be an appropriate way of offering help to both Paul and his contemporaries.

The initial contract was a simple one. The worker promised to be at a certain place in the project for one and a half hours at the same time each week. Paul made the same commitment. It was the least painful way of satisfying his probation officer. He was encouraged to let his friends know that the worker was available to whomever showed up. The worker would help organize various athletic games and before long there were fifteen to twenty boys attending "the group." Although called "the group" by the worker, there was at this point no sense of a group process other than consistent attention from a man. This was an acceptable level of treatment at this point. Basic reliability and trust were being established in a safe context. During this time there were relatively few conflicts.

When the numbers attending became unmanageable it was apparent that there was a need for changes that would address some issues of beginning commitment or preaffiliation. The agency provided additional leaders and suggested a split in the group by age. The boys managed a split into "big kids" (12-13) and "little kids" (10-12). This process was largely controlled by the participants and arrived at by consensus of all present.

From this point we will follow the "big kids" group, now with male co-leaders. The contract and process had begun to change in that the boys now saw themselves as logically selected members of an entity called "the group." Attendance was still loose and membership remained open. However, attendance had become more consistent, and the boys began to notice absences. The level of commitment to each other had increased. This separation into smaller groups was the first opportunity to create a sense of group identity. It had also introduced a method for dealing with group matters: members would be given a great deal of control, and a general consensus would be followed. Perhaps most significant, the leaders were more available to the smaller number.

The group, on its own initiative, began to leave the project area during group time, and began to expand their repertoire of activities. At the same time the workers increased their commitment and clearly stated a new contract. The workers would now provide transportation and a small amount of money, fifty cents per boy, as a base for expanding activities. The commitment on the part of the boys was concurrently expanded to include appropriate behavior in the car and community. They also agreed that the money would be used to help the group in its activities, and would not be used for anything outside of group. The decisions about activities were to be in the group's hands, and would be reached by unanimous decision.

If this were an in-house group, or a group with more motivation for change, the workers would have been looking for activities designed to help the process of affiliation. These would have encouraged interaction while allowing distance, providing physical safety and enhancing self-esteem. The workers would have provided a good deal of program structure, introducing activities that minimized frustration and competitive interaction while ensuring initial satisfaction and success (Garland et al., p. 42). Middleman suggests an approach to programs where the leader(s) carefully plans, carries out, and analyzes each activity. The leader(s) consider purpose, content, skill demanded, surrounding conditions, and transition to the next activity (pp. 141-145).

These are all very important issues to the success of an activity and therefore of the activity group. However, we must also consider the population involved. These boys' behavior, while troublesome to the community, was syntonic, both individually and as a peer group. They had tremendous difficulty with authorities. Anger and testing behaviors played themselves out in many of their relationships. For the most part they were eager for a relationship with the workers, but they were ready to do battle with them as well. The major goal in this early phase was to avoid getting caught in control struggles. It would have been a losing battle. The predictable results would be self-defeating; an aborted group effort, increased alienation of the youths, a sense of failure for agency and workers, and resignation that these are indeed untreatable young people. Having realized this, the question became, what controls do the leaders need to establish, and what controls are best given to the membership.

We saw a pattern develop to deal with authority and control issues in the splitting of the group and in choosing activities. Now the horizons of the group were broadened by use of a car and money. These additions heightened potential power struggles. The leaders owned the car(s) and were literally in the driver's seat. They were the holders and providers of money, which embodies real and symbolic power as the sustenance of the group. This power and control was managed so as not to provoke self-defeating struggles. This was accomplished in ways consistent with the emerging process.

It was made clear that the money was provided by the agency, not a personal gift. It would not be awarded or withheld based on behavior; it was a given part of the agency commitment. Decisions about how to spend the money were left to the members, again on a unanimous basis. The leaders distributed money once the decision was made. Naturally this stimulated control battles among members, but very little with the leaders. The limited amount was objected to at times, but the group was encouraged to supplement it.

This process was not so easily accomplished with the workers' cars. There was not the freedom to make this a given at all times. The car itself, the people in it, and others on the road had to be protected. The limits around use of the car had to be clearly stated and fairly enforced. They were certainly tested. Use of the car was not withheld when the leaders were unhappy with the group, nor was it used in a manipulative fashion to limit the choices given to the group. No matter what the group may have done to anger or frustrate the leaders, the use of the car was limited only when appropriately related to abuse of the car.

The mobility provided by the car also presented related difficulties in terms of behavior in the community. Again the contract was expanding with a parallel need for agreement on limits. As few rules as possible were used so that testing would occur in controlled ways. The rules were chosen to be clearly acceptable to the group, while covering the needs of the workers. The only hard and fast rules were that behavior stay within the law, and that it was not acceptable to hurt people or damage property.

Another important factor was the attitude of the workers. The oppositional behavior typical for these boys must be viewed in an objective way. It is a common trap to get one's ego caught up in suggesting or completing activities. Flexibility is important in all groups and most important in this kind of group. The leader(s) can ''not give up and feel personally rejected if the group does not want to go along with him'' (Middleman, pp. 140-141).

With this group most suggestions of the leaders were rejected as the ''shrinks' '' agenda, and it became clear that a carefully preplanned program was not workable. A more reactive style had to be developed. Rather than analyzing and designing a specific program, the workers used activities suggested by the group members. Of course, within the process of suggestion and decision there was much latitude, and it was in this area that the leaders could function most effectively. Program decisions were based on what would be the most fun thing to do on a given day and how powerful was the proponent of that activity. We would accept, within bounds, the activity selection made by the group so long as they were able to work it out unanimously. Sometimes the activity made sense in terms of group development, sometimes it did not. However, a significant process for decision making had been introduced. It provided acceptable program to the boys and avoided major control struggles between leaders and members. As much as possible could be done with the activity regardless of its appropriateness. The leaders would still analyze the activity and when appropriate share this with the group. This involved raising concerns, pointing out and facilitating difficulties in the decision making, and being willing to help the group in controlling itself. Limits were almost always acceptable to the group in this context so long as they made sense in a concrete way.

The method of program selection and decision making that evolved worked because of its somewhat paradoxical nature. Confrontation was avoided by saying in effect, "It's up to you guys what we do," rather than, "Here's an activity like it or not." The twist came in how this was then carried out. The leaders were very active in insisting that a program selection be reached by the agreed upon method. This had the effect of saying, "We are going to make *you* decide what *you* want to do," always thrusting it back in their laps. The leaders were acting in behalf, almost as the protectors and keepers, of the members' control. The leaders would make sure that no one violated this control: leaders, members or outsiders. When limits had to be set, this also was deflected into the agreed upon group process. For example, acting-out might be addressed as follows: "The group has decided to go to the bowling alley, but it seems we cannot carry out this plan due to specific behavior. Does the group want to follow through with its own program?" Again, note the importance of the leaders not being heavily invested in that program.

Pre-affiliation

During pre-affiliation the most popular activities were: eating (mostly at MacDonalds), sports (unlike in the outreach phase, now member initiated), bowling alley (bowling, pool, pinball machines and food), going to the zoo, and cruising in the car. Most of the sports activities fit nicely into our goals. The major sport was floor hockey. This entailed advance planning as the gym space and equipment had to be arranged ahead of time. There was plenty of room for interaction and cooperation, but it was also all right to sit out or play separately. Cruising was a very difficult activity for the group to manage. It was a very intimate situation. Everyone was packed into a crowded car, legs touching. There were many references to homosexuality. The leaders attempted to turn cruising into a transitional activity, by the inclusion of a destination. The bowling alley was an activity that allowed distance but was too seductive to promote whole group interaction. This would usually turn into a subgroup experience with some people playing pool, some bowling, some eating, and some playing pinball.

The group's behavior and level of development at this point

would have excluded some of these from the leaders' list of preferred activities. However, these were the group's decisions, and key issues were raised in spite of, sometimes because of, occasional inability to complete the activity as planned. These situations provided opportunities to get them thinking about group process. Each member's impact on the group became clear when all members had to stop and leave due to the ejection of one member by outside authorities. The group had decided on the activity, the group had to deal with its failure. An example was the group's frequent choice of visiting the zoo. We had to stop when it became clear that Bob could not keep himself from abusing the animals. This was not an ideal activity for this stage, but that didn't make sense to the group until Bob demonstrated why. However, going to the zoo became a goal for the group.

Power and Control

Once the group became fairly consistent in membership, testing took on a different quality. Acting-out in the car, unsafe and destructive behavior, reached a point where we had to limit the use of the car fairly often. Competition for shot-gun (the front window seat) became fierce, the normal development of a group's need to test the limits of the group, the leaders, and each other. At this point we would ideally structure activities that allow this process to happen in acceptable ways. We would look for activities that required low planning, that could tolerate program breakdown, and that would include aggressive competition. We would allow the testing of strength and authority (Garland et al., pp. 42-46). Because the choice of activities rested with the group, the program during this period was not designed with these issues in mind. Again the bowling alley and eating were popular, as were occasional attempts to get us to the zoo. This was a predictably difficult time for the group to decide on or plan activities, and it was even more difficult for them to accept suggestions from the leaders. Thus, the activity for the day might be to fight over a choice. The leaders in keeping the group to the decision making process, were able to permit rebellion, protect the safety of individuals and property, and work at clarifying the struggle (Garland et al., pp. 42-46).

Perhaps the clearest illustration of reactive group building during this difficult time was a day when we were not allowing use of the car. The group was angry and stuck for an activity. The leaders offered many suggestions for activities that did not include the use of the automobile. The group was immobilized. They began in a passive and sullen way, but ended in a loud cohesive chorus with, "Aw, shut up," following each suggestion we made. This response was allowed, the leaders in fact encouraged it by continuing to come up with new ideas, until this game became the activity. The group was more together than it had ever been. Many such struggles occurred over a long time. They were seen as an important part of the group's development rather than roadblocks. In this case the leaders had taken a seemingly fruitless struggle and used the group's anger to create a productive and, in the end, fun activity.

A number of conflicts at this time were related to membership. Members and leaders increasingly verbalized the presence or absence of specific boys. Members did some of their own outreach to new or absent boys. Control battles were most intense around inclusion/exclusion and ranking. Again the leaders tried not to get entrapped in these confrontations, and worked to foster a sense of process and group decision making. Thus, if one boy was being excluded, the leaders would try to bring the conflict to the attention of the entire group. A good example of ranking occurred when Al entered the group. As a new member Al had low status, although his status in the community was high. The group was stuck in making any program decision. Al decided to take the lead, announced we were walking to the corner store, and set off at a brisk pace, only to look back and see everyone sitting still. He returned and this effort was repeated a number of times. Al's rank at this point was so low that he never recovered, dropped out soon after, and successfully found a non-delinquent peer group. Without interfering in what was actually happening, the leaders clarified this process both for Al and the group.

During this stage the leaders also made a point of reiterating their own and the group's responsibility to ensure safety. Physical interaction was often intense. Important issues of self-control arose weekly. Serious fighting occurred outside of group time on several occasions. These events were used as opportunities to expand the contract. Although reluctant at first, the group tolerated bringing such outside events into the group for discussion and resolution.

Intimacy

As the power and control issues settled down a comfortable more intimate tone emerged. Fluctuation in membership decreased, the group being a steady six to eight members. The members still had the power of activity selection, but their selections reflected a sense of group identity and mutuality. They were interested in visiting motorcycle shops, staying together to share enthusiasm. They also worked out the problems around visiting the zoo. Bob could respond to the group's pressure and control his angry impulses. Cruising, which had been too intense at an earlier point, was now relaxed and enjoyable. They were still interested in eating, but now would get pizza and bring it to the agency to eat, play board games, or talk. They shared concerns about each other's self-destructive and anti-social behavior. This included working out ways to re-involve a depressed and drug dependent member, and constructively help another who had run away from home but was attending the group. Insight that would be unacceptable "shrink" talk if presented by the leaders, grew out of some of these discussions. For example, in talking about stealing and getting arrested, the leaders participated, but in a low key nonjudgmental way. It was one of the members, after a lengthy discussion of numerous incidents, who finally said, "You know, I think we want to be caught."

Garland et al. suggest that this is a time when program can be openly emotion laden, and struggles for attention and material can be anticipated. The stakes are higher now. There is a growing ability to plan and carry out projects, but often with emotional turmoil (pp. 51-52). In this group the leaders did not have to plan these programs. The group decided on very intimate kinds of activities, accepting and even joining the workers in processing group experiences. The high point of this development was the use of Shephard Brooks, a nearby conservation area. The group first chose to go there during the Power and Control stage and used the opportunity to run away from the leaders. The response turned this behavior into a legitimate game of hide and seek. As time and cohesiveness progressed this game became a very elaborate group ritual. The members' refinements included such things as the use of walkie-talkies.

The central meeting place at Shephard Brooks was a grotto-like area called "The Rock," which became the group's "office." They would refuse to discuss anything until we got to "The Rock" at which time they would be capable of the deepest, most intimate discussions. Even though we had progressed this far as a group they needed to keep their vestiges of control. If we tried to talk in the car about an issue, they would shut us up saying, "Wait until we get to

The Rock!'' They could now manage this easily and relate the issues discussed to the rest of their life experience.

Membership also underwent a significant change. As the group grew closer entry became more closed, and a formal application procedure was established. Rules for guests, for trying out the group, for bringing a potential member, were mutually agreed upon. The most sophisticated part of this was a written application to be completed by a new member with a youth worker in the housing project office. This was a significant step in the group's seeing itself as part of a community wide program.

Differentiation

In Differentiation, as in Intimacy, the leaders did not have to work hard at productive uses of inappropriate activities. The group was running smoothly. Members were giving to each other freely, including a sharing of roles. There were well developed traditions and customs. Activities were cooperative and complex projects were undertaken. Outside interests became more important and the group was able to act as a unit in relation to the community (Garland et al., pp. 52-56).

Activities included a continuation of the Shephard Brooks rituals and the formation of a committee to deal with the Public Housing Authority. The natural peer group of boys had been at odds with the Housing Authority since their pre-teen years. (They were now sixteen.) At issue was the lack of a legitimate place for the boys to hang around and socialize. Traditionally they would hang on someone's porch until they were moved, by a neighbor or the police. Conflict was frequent. They were now at an age and size where people were more fearful of them and wanted them moved once and for all. There was, however, no alternative place for them to gather and they responded to pressure by increased acting-out behavior.

They were able to discuss this conflict in the group and managed to act as a committee that would attend Housing Authority meetings and make well thought out and documented proposals for a gathering spot. They sold their idea to the Tenant's Association and to the Housing Authority, including a commitment to policing themselves and the area. This was a long, frustrating struggle. The leaders were helpful in this process, but the activity was the group's. Again, there was little divergence in goals. We also see here a significant pay-off of group work in achieving streetwork objectives. Without flexibility and the group base it would have been impossible to complete this project.

Separation

It became evident the group was moving into the final stage when we began to hear more about getting jobs, spending time with a girl friend, or working on a car; all conflicting with group time. One member was planning to enter the service. There were considerable ups and downs as the boys began to move out in these directions. The movement was steady, the members taking the lead, and still using the group as a support.

In order to facilitate a healthy separation, the leaders needed to take a more directive position. It was time to help the group bring itself to a logical and positive conclusion lest it fall apart amidst boredom, confused loyalties and guilt. Attendance was inconsistent, with a few core members angry at the lack of commitment. The work on the gathering spot was done and the suggested activities were stale. We were in a rut but the members were too invested in the group to suggest any substantive changes. The message finally got through to the leaders one week when no one was at the meeting spot. Instead, a messenger was sent to tell us that the group was together but they had forgotten it was group day and had gotten high. Being aware of the rule about being under the influence of drugs in group, they were sending their regrets and would see us the following week. For the workers this incident symbolized a regression as well as a beginning process of recapitulation. It was the potential beginning of what Garland et al. refer to as nihilistic flight (p. 61).

The leaders began to interpret the groups stuck position and to reframe it in terms of the positive progression of the group experience. We spent a good deal of time clarifying for them that this was, in fact, the way groups work and that they appeared to have met the goals of the group. We stated clearly that we felt it was time to look at the history of the group, in terms of these goals, and come to a decision together about ending.

This was a long process that involved considerable resistance. The immediate reaction was one of denial. "We don't have to end the group." "So what if only one or two people come." This represented a pseudo-acceptance of regression in the level of commitment. They were frightened of letting go of important relationships and experiences that had been consistent throughout their adolescent years. Another response was the feeling of rejection. One boy said, ''Why don't you just drive us back to the projects and forget you ever knew us?'' We assured them of the workers' and the agency's continued commitment to each of them and our availability to them in other ways, but stuck to the obvious diminishing returns and completed goals.

We had to actively stay with this position as the boys were insistent about their wish and need to continue. ''How about if we start doing B & Es (breaking and entering) again? That will show you that we need the group.'' All of these protestations were unaccompanied by renewed commitment or more consistent attendance. The leaders supported their other commitments, but pointed out that the group was too important to allow it to simply fade away. We continually reinforced the idea that the five year group could be terminated in a very positive way so that everyone could feel they had completed an important and rewarding experience.

We planned a few meetings to look specifically at the history and goals of the group as a way of measuring its success and need for continuation. These meetings, in and of themselves, represented the success of the group. In the beginning stages the only goals the members could identify were, ''to have fun,'' and, ''to keep us out of trouble.'' They could listen to our goals for them but could express no investment in them. Now they participated eagerly in drawing up a list of what they had grown to see as goals for the group. One member wrote them on a blackboard:

1. Keep out of trouble.
2. Some sort of counseling.
3. To have fun.
4. Face a problem as a group.
5. Learn to get along with other people
   a. with adults
   b. with associates
   c. with community
6. Take different roles

Each contribution led to a lively discussion of examples in the group's history and to an increased awareness of their growth and development as a group. The members became invested in evaluating and insisted that the list of goals be preserved for the next meeting by writing on the board in their strongest terms, "LEAVE THE FUCK ALONE." Termination was beginning to feel acceptable to them.

During this period we also allowed and encouraged a repetition of many of the successful and some of the unsuccessful activities in the group's history. They had a very different flavor this time around. Some of the old testing behavior resurfaced but was much more easily dealt with and could be used as a way for the group to measure its own growth. Cruising in the car served as a time to reminisce. Visiting the zoo provided the opportunity to remember how the group had helped Bob control his impulses. This also brought up how important everyone felt the group had been in helping Bob with his depression and drug abuse. The boys were suggesting activities in order to remember and rework old issues. Their readiness to terminate was clear when a special hiding place at Shephard Brooks was finally revealed to the leaders in the next to last meeting. It was a secret that they ceremoniously wanted the whole group to share before ending.

The final meeting was a party that had been planned by the group as a celebration. As their "gift" to us they once again showed their high level of organization and cohesiveness. They had planned comprehensive ways of testing out all the old limits, "For old time's sake." Beer was smuggled into the agency. Food was played with in a pro forma manner. One of the boys lit up a joint in the car, forcing us to stop and deal with the infraction. These all provided us the opportunity to interpret the behavior in terms of the termination process, and it gave the boys a chance to make sure we still cared about them. This testing behavior was, in fact, more symbolic than acting-out. One of the boys made sure that we were aware of the significance of their choice of beverage, Lowenbrau, which was advertising itself at the time, "Here's to good friends, tonight is kinda special . . ."

The prognosis for all these boys had been poor. The group was not a cure for all their individual and peer pathologies, but a significant impact was made. They sustained a therapeutic experience for five years, being seventeen when we ended. It is clear this would not have happened had we invited them into the agency to change their social functioning. The group gave them a more flexible, positive and hopeful view of themselves and life. It has helped move them into new interests and healthier functioning. This intervention represents a considerable agency commitment, but an effective one in reaching alienated youth and providing a level of group experience generally thought to be out of their reach.

REFERENCES

Bernstein, S. *Youth on the Streets.* New York: Association Press, 1964.

Garland, J. A., Jones, H. E., and Kolodny, R. A. A Model for Stages of Development in Social Group Work. In S. Bernstein (Ed.), *Explorations in Group Work.* Boston: Milford House Inc., 1973.

Middleman, R. R. *The Non-Verbal Method in Working with Groups.* Hebron Conn.: Practitioners' Press Inc., 1980.

Television Production as Content and Process in Social Work with Groups: An Experiment with Disadvantaged Neighborhood Youth in Israel

Dov Shinar

ABSTRACT. Closed circuit television was utilized to improve the application of social work with groups to disadvantaged neighborhood youth. A workshop was conducted with a youth group, where members learned to use video techniques and produced programs concerning personal and social problems. Evaluation included participant observation and analysis of videotape recordings.

The findings identify group processes, including Tuckman's sequential development stages, indicate therapeutic and social community effects, and help validate the unique characteristics of social work with groups. They suggest that while the group was a necessary condition, television production—as process and content—provided the sufficient condition for change to occur. Comparative analysis of television and other group activities indicate the advantages of the former in social work with groups.

The activation of neighborhood groups, which has served in recent years as an intervention approach with disadvantaged youth in Israel, has encountered severe difficulties in the development of values, attitudes and skills. In spite of the relative effectiveness in the instrumental domain, social workers have seen few positive results in the treatment of intellectual underdevelopment, lack of self-confidence, objective and subjective alienation (the "outcast complex"), low motivation, juvenile delinquency, and high dropout rates from school and jobs. Previous experience with the use of closed circuit television suggested that its application could offer

Dov Shinar is Communications Coordinator, Brookdale Institute of Gerontology and Adult Human Development, J.D.C. Hill, P.O.B. 13087, Jerusalem, 91130 Israel.

ways to cope with some of these problems as well as contribute to the general theory and practice of social work with groups.

Video and Social Action

The process of "re-inventing" television, so as to make it more relevant to society (Kalba, 1974), has been characterized in the last decade by the growing use of video technology for the treatment of social problems. In addition to its utilization for training and therapy, experimental work with closed circuit television suggests the applicability of its structure and process to social work with groups and youth, adult education, community development, social action and cross-cultural communication.

Videotape "narrowcasting" is free from most limitations imposed on broadcasting by its institutional, economic, technical and aesthetic structure. Such constraints limit the amount and types of subjects dealt with by professional television, make production inaccessible to the public (Elliott, 1972), and do not allow "reciprocal action between transmitter and receiver . . ." thus "reduc(ing) feedback to the lowest point compatible with the system" (Enzesberger, 1972, p. 101).

Closed circuit television is characterized by flexibility, openness to wide participation, ease of operation, immediacy of feedback and review, relatively low cost, and convenience of display and distribution (Casey, 1974; Atienza, 1977; Stuart, 1977; Mott, 1979). The resulting structure allows for ". . . zeroing in on particular problems, communities and constituencies," stressing "a process rather than a product . . . oriented toward problem-solving activities" (Ingle, 1974, p. 20). Its participatory nature, perhaps, provides the possibility of fulfilling Brecht's (1932) declared design to change radio (and all electronic media, for that matter) from a means of distribution into a means of communication.

Accounts of the use of closed circuit television in work with groups mention a variety of methods and processes, ranging from "active exposure" to televised contents (Rhodes Center, 1970; Shinar, 1972), to participation in processs of production, distribution and reception (Ingle, 1974; Tannenbaum, 1976; VED, 1979). These methods have been employed to change the attitudes of and activate urban and rural communities (Kennedy, 1973; Schultz, 1974; Thenot, 1979), as well as to work with specific groups and problems. Examples include tenants' rights in low income neighborhoods, youth unemployment, family violence, rehabilitation of jail inmates (VED, 1979), inter-religious dialogue (Access, 1973), and problems with the aged (Tannenbaum, 1976). The reported results of these experiments mention the effectiveness of closed circuit television in developing teamwork, in planning and delaying gratification, in encouraging and improving decision making, creating expression, performance skills and continuous effort, and in intensifying relationships with the immediate and external environment.

The Experiment

Following these premises, an experiment was conducted with the objective of assessing the effects of participation in closed circuit television production on a neighborhood youth group. Its purpose was to alleviate problems in such crucial areas as awareness of self and of social image, relations with the environment, and lack of important skills and attitudes. The experiment, carried out jointly by the Jerusalem Municipality's Division for Youth Advancement and the Hebrew University's Division for Communications in Education, was undertaken with a neighborhood youth group of 12 members (10 males and 2 females). With varying membership, the group had been active for almost two years.

The neighborhood, with a population of about 30,000, was founded in 1968. At the time of the experiment it was populated with new immigrants, including a large number of elderly persons, and with disadvantaged families transferred from other problem-ridden neighborhoods. The new housing, wide roads and good public buildings stood in contrast with the neighborhood's inadequate services and problematic community organization. The physical and cultural atmosphere soon deteriorated. Neither the older nor younger generations took pride in their neighborhood, which developed a culture of poverty—not necessarily in the economic sense.

The group members, aged 15-18, consisted of eleven second-generation Israelis and one new immigrant. Four members came from families where the father was chronically ill or unemployed. The majority lived under circumstances of economic constraint. All members worked and some went to evening school. Dropping out and changing jobs, however, was common practice and a number of them had minor delinquency records.

In order to formulate the experiment's design and procedure, a half-day meeting of the group was organized, during which the participants visited the University studios and were given the opportunity to operate the equipment and watch recordings of their work. Analysis of the preliminary session suggested that this type of activity could stimulate and motivate the participants, could develop critical abilities towards self and others (especially when watching recorded images), and could have a strong social impact, as expressed in the participants' pride in visiting the University and being trusted with the operation of expensive equipment.

Consequently, a decision was made to conduct an eight-month workshop with supervised group discussions, practical training and field practice, as well as independent sub-group and individual work. The staff included a project director experienced in the application of television in formal and informal education, a senior social worker experienced in neighborhood treatment, two field coordinators (the neighborhood group's permanent social worker and a media instruction worker), three television instructors, and one evaluation worker.

The procedure started in the neighborhood. Following the group members' request for a second visit to the studios, the social worker's suggestion to organize a closed-circuit television production workshop was accepted by the members. The formal goal was program production upon completion of which the members would be given proper credit.

Work began with a weekly meeting at the University facilities, including a twenty minute introductory period, followed by an hour of practical training, and a second half-hour discussion period. During the introductory period, short explanations were given of television work and production exercises were explored and analyzed. The practical work included equipment operation (cameras, sound, lighting, editing, control), production elements (subject research, scriptwriting, interviewing and aesthetic guidance (directing, staging, etc.). The group visited Israel Television, where they met and talked with "colleagues" and conducted production exercises at prestigious sites, such as the Jerusalem Theater.

Most of the discussion periods were devoted to the exploration of the production subjects, possible approaches, and means of gathering information. Such discussions served to assess attitudes, "weak spots," and common concerns. The subjects were selected after eight meetings and included: (1) youth problems in the neighborhood, (2) jobs held by group members, and (3) juvenile delinquen-cy. The participants divided into three sub-groups by program sub-jects selected and during the next six months met twice a week for supervised and independent work on their projects. This part of the workshop took place in the neighborhood and was conducted in ad-dition to the weekly group meeting. Each sub-group planned and produced a 10-15 minute program, including its creative and tech-nical components. They were advised and guided by the staff on equipment operation and the definition of problems, but seldom on solutions.

Closed circuit television also served as an evaluation device. The workshop meetings were openly videotaped by staff and participants (as a practical exercise). The material was analyzed and served as part of the data for this report.

Of the ten boys and two girls who participated in the workshop, four left before the conclusion of the work. At the end, the par-ticipants invited parents, staff and friends to a party at the Universi-ty. The programs were screened with the accompaniment of pro-ducers' presentations. Diplomas were given and speeches made by the participants and the staff.

Group Processes

Tuckman's conceptualization (1965) of changes in structure and activity of different group settings—therapy, training, natural and laboratory groups—suggests a sequential development, with stages applicable to this group. The "forming" stage consisted of group orientation, identification of inter-personal and task boundaries, and development of dependency relationships. This phase occurred dur-ing the initial eight weeks. The participants at first tried to use the workshop as a means for immediate personal gratification. The struggles to operate one of the three cameras or to hold a microphone and serve as the interviewer, imitating popular televi-sion personalities, were expressions of these feelings. The at-mosphere changed as participants were required to perform more complicated tasks, such as plugging together the technical systems, serving as interviewers, and analyzing the televised feedback. The participants began to recognize their difficulties in verbal expression and in making orderly translations of ideas into visual terms. A pro-cess of self and mutual discovery and evaluation began at this stage, which included the identification of the participants' relative task performance skills and the development of a competition-cooperation continuum of interaction.

Professional intervention during the initial stage consisted of setting general ground rules, as required by the university environment, by the equipment, and by the dynamics of the group situation. Technical instruction was provided, along with assistance in the formulation of production projects and inconspicuous special help to the weaker participants.

Tuckman's second sequence point, "storming," consists of "conflict and polarization around interpersonal issues with concomitant emotional responding in the task sphere" (p. 346). In the group, this phase started with the division into sub-groups according to the production topics. Typically, competition and hostility developed with respect to personal, sub-group and group issues and prevailed over 7-8 weeks.

Large gaps appeared between the unrealistic aspirations expressed in the subject selection and participants' actual abilities and the constraints inherent in the process. Stronger participants lacked tolerance toward the others. The two sub-groups which made slower progress expressed frustration and despair, often in the form of a fatalistic attitude, ascribing failure to "the curse on our lives." The more successful sub-group demanded all the project staff's attention. Some members left the workshop, unable to cope with criticism and tension; however, several returned at the request of friends. Guidance, planning and evaluation meetings became almost impossible, to the point of endangering the workshop's continuation.

The situation of conflict and the resulting increase in aggressiveness found two external outlets, in addition to its impact on group cohesiveness. The first outlet consisted of hostile reactions to the videotaping of the meetings for evaluation purposes. Opposition to the recordings, which was not expressed in the beginning, became a controversial issue between participants and staff. In addition to serving as an outlet for tensions and frustrations typical of this phase, the reaction reflected fears of outside exposure, anxieties over feelings of manipulation, and a refusal to let others participate in the experience. The second external manifestation consisted of aggressiveness towards the environment, which stood in striking contrast with the acceptance of the basic ground rules set for the workshop. Although the participants never tried to harm the equipment and always behaved responsibly during the sessions, their exit through the university buildings and bus ride home were always violent during this phase. It ranged from aggressive shouting and quarreling, to kicking trash containers, to slamming doors, etc. These reactions were displayed by all the participants, regardless of their positions in the group situation.

Intervention at this phase consisted of discussions at the interpersonal, sub-group and group levels. Emphasis was placed on the need to establish a clear contractual relationship among the participants and between the group and the staff. Recognition was given to the equal rights of all participants and emphasis placed on the group process nature of television production in the workshop. Psychological reinforcement, such as video demonstrations of each member's behavior, visits to Israel Television's studios, and talks with professionals helped to clarify these points. The process was slow and painful, but the wish to continue the production finally prevailed over frustration and lack of confidence.

"Norming," the third stage identified by Tuckman, is characterized by growing cohesiveness, the expression of intimate relationships, and the development of standards and new roles. It occurred in the group during the next 3-4 weeks.

Insofar as group activity was concerned, the previous wild individual and sub-group competition gradually changed to various types and degrees of cooperation within and between sub-groups, a development encouraged by the staff. Mutual assistance began to show up in areas where certain participants excelled, such as camera work, interviewing, planning and organization, regardless of sub-group allegiance. As this process provided answers to production problems and contributed to recognizable progress, tensions and frustrations were gradually replaced by rational planning.

Norming in regard to the environment was expressed in several directions. First, the groups accepted the staff's firm stand on continued recording of the sessions for evaluation pruposes. Their acceptance was based on the staff's explanations about the necessity of learning from this first, innovative experiment. The development of agreed upon rules relied on involvement with the equipment and its demands. In the "forming" and "storming" stages, the prohibition on smoking in the studios disrupted the meetings, as participants left the room in order to smoke and created continuous movement. In the "norming" phase, smoking breaks were introduced, which became less and less frequent as time went by. The disorderly behavior on university premises decreased as the participants began to feel more at ease and to see themselves as a legitimate part of the system. Intervention at this stage consisted of the prevention of disruption and encouraging the development of group consciousness.

Tuckman's fourth stage—"performing"—integrates the resolution of previous structural problems and the channeling of group energy into task performance. This was characteristic of the last three months in the life of the group. The participants employed the skills and lessons they learned to produce their programs. Research and planning were completed, scripts were written and evaluated by the entire group, the work on location and in the studios was done, sound tracks were recorded, graphics and captions prepared, and the final editing process took place. These activities were typically performed with disregard for conventional working hours and with considerable effort. The participants came up with original and surprising ideas, shot fairly good visual segments, and later edited them into logical and sensitive, although amateurish, sequences.

The programs were screened at a last session, in which criticism was put forth and accepted almost on professional grounds. The formal screening, during the final party with families and staff, made some of the achievements even clearer. The youths made both prepared and improvised speeches which gave rich and concise verbal expression to their experience. This stood in complete contrast with the initial phases, when the participants were unable to express their ideas coherently.

The Products

The youth's work on their television programs produced (1) therapeutic effects, and (2) social community effects at both individual and group levels. These effects are clearly expressed in the follow-up videotapes and the staff's written records. Individual therapeutic effects included behavioral changes which affected all the participants, increased self-confidence and self-esteem, and the change of an initially fatalistic approach to one of relating analysis, planning, and learning to the solution of problems. Two examples are particularly outstanding.

The first refers to a youth who at the time the workshop began found himself at a crossroads. Frustrated with his daily life, he contemplated engaging in delinquent activity as an easy way to satisfy his aspirations. Unable to reach a decision, due to opposing internalized values, he was in deep self-conflict and had severe functional difficulties. Being highly intelligent and having leadership qualities, he used the workshop as an outlet and had his sub-group select juvenile-delinquency as their research topic. During the research and program recording the boy interviewed ex-criminals, police and probation officers, with the double purpose of using the information for his own needs. After completing the program, he confided to the social worker his awareness of the double purpose and explained it by his wish not to expose himself and to preserve a positive image.

The second case was that of one of the girls who, due to a lack of self-confidence, did not dare to say a single work during the discussions of the first five months. At most, she whispered to her girl friend. When production was already well underway, she slowly began to express her views and opinions to the point that during the last eight weeks she exerted a stabilizing influence on the group through public expression and practical assistance given to others.

Therapeutic effects at another level were found in the group's conclusion that even complex tasks could be accomplished through teamwork and that contractual relationships and mutual responsibility pay off in terms of group solidarity. Thus, the process, which started with a group concept that perceived only individual and technical tasks, developed to include established procedures of mutual assistance and cohesiveness.

Social-community effects at the individual level included a significant improvement in verbal, written and other types of expression, which contributed to increased individual self-confidence and to group functioning. Whether in phrasing interview questions, writing scripts, or presenting their programs, progress could be seen in the participants' communication abilities.

The social-community effects at the group level appeared in increased involvement with the community and higher group status. The workshop participants interviewed and talked to residents of their neighborhood, including business people, service agents, officials, housewives, and children. The professional attitude and poise demonstrated by the group during the program production impressed the neighborhood residents, contributed to the group's status and consequently to their self-esteem. The feeling of acceptance by the "legitimate" environment, represented by the University, television "colleagues" and others, made a definite contribution to these effects. At least they realized that the environment was not totally hostile.

Discussion

The effects described in the previous section, make it clear that the method employed gave feasible answers to difficulties of self-awareness and image, to problematic relationships with the internal and external environments, and to the lack of certain functional values, attitudes and skills. Obviously, the duration of these effects and methods of increasing the cost-effectiveness are subjects for further inquiry, but the results seem encouraging.

The conclusions also concern methodology, particularly in helping to depict the unique qualities of social work with groups, as compared to group therapy and other types of group treatment. In a recent analysis of the relevant literature, Lang sets forth a number of criteria to make a distinction among these approaches. She also stresses the lack of empirical evidence necessary "to move beyond abstract model conceptualizations to a clear operational specification of practice technology" (1979b, p. 205). The present experiment attempts to bring empirical validation to her criteria.

(1) A full fledged social group, rather than "a psychological collectivity" (Lang, 1979, p. 210), was featured as the central entity. The group functioned not in terms of a symbolic collectivity, such as frequently appears in group therapies, but as an authentic social reality. The workshop admittedly did include some symbolic elements, such as the creation of sub-groups and the aspects of play involved in the process. In contrast, however, to group therapies, where some elements are highly artificial, symbols appeared in the workshop as valid expressions of group life. The sub-groups were composed according to members' choices within the context of common intra-group goals; and the play elements stemmed from the group and were instrumental to its work. (2) Even under the constraints imposed by the requirements of television work, interaction was natural and spontaneous, free from the highly controlled and constricted process typical of group therapies. The interaction was an authentic expression of the group, instrumental in the processing of its goals (Tropp, 1977) and transferable to other parts of members' lives, not a self-conscious scrutiny. (3) In contrast to the typical linear therapist-patient relationships, the route to change proceeded through the process mentioned by Lang (1979b, p. 213) as a merging of self with others in collective, integrated undertakings, along a non-linear path. Instead of treatment by an expert, which often interferes with individual privacy, staff activities emphasized

social functioning and links between the individual, group, and environment. The professionals' role was conceived as participation in and contribution to the group process, so as to increase its potential for serving the intended ends of members, while simultaneously respecting the boundaries and autonomy of both individual and group (Lang, 1979b; Heap, 1979). The experiment displayed multidimensional, complex and subtle means of growth and change, in contrast with the specific, direct and explicit techniques of group therapies.

Further conclusions concern the role of television production in social work with groups. The findings indicate that the group was the major agent of change. One could contend, however, that the group functioned only as a necessary condition; whereas television— both as process and as content—provided the sufficient condition, without which change could not be achieved. The findings on the individual and social effects of television production seem to support this contention with reference to process. Moreover, the findings tend to confirm previous experience, that groups do not always have sufficient internal "content resources" to encourage change and that social workers are not always successful in developing such resources (Lang, 1979b). Television work and play, both in front and behind cameras and monitors, provided such content directly and stimulated the development of latent resources.

Admittedly, television production is not the only possible activity in work with groups. Drama and sports are good examples of alternative activities. Television production does seem to have advantages in "supporting and facilitating interaction even when the members are at deficit in their social skills . . ." (Lang, 1979b, p. 213) and of playing a significant part in the group's formation development and functioning (Rosenthal, 1973). Television production appears to be sufficiently specific to develop and maintain groups' cohesiveness and broad enough to accommodate individual inclinations, abilities and limitations. The present experience supports Piccardo's experience with film (1974). Unlike sports or drama, media production reduces competitiveness and encourages cooperation. Furthermore, television production offers a wide range of aesthetic, technical, organizational and other roles, and thus is less alienating than sports or drama, which are more selective and tend to limit participation to the more talented, inclined or able.

In addition, the elements of task and play are better balanced in television production. Like sports or drama, the process involves a considerable amount of play and symbolic activity which contributes to its effectiveness in developing motivation. But unlike these activities, which are entirely symbolic, the findings on the use of video production as a means of social activation indicate greater effectiveness in the replication of reality and its demands (Willener, 1976). Video production was found to encourage the injection of subjective experience into reality, along with rational observation, thus stimulating the creative discovery of self and environment (see Vincelli, 1975; Rosler, 1977). In our experience the process and content of closed circuit television production are highly applicable to the requirements of effective social work with groups (Lang, 1979b), especially concerning inter-personal connections among group members and the mobilization of group strengths in relation to the environment (Pattison, 1965; Mallinson, 1965). Television production allows for consideration to group composition and provides for easy activation and development of group identity.

BIBLIOGRAPHY AND REFERENCES

Access, VTR in Cross Cultural Communications. *Challenge for Change.* Montreal: National Film Board of Canada, Spring 1973, 20-21.
Atienza, L. *VTR Workshop Small Format Video.* Paris, UNESCO, 1977.
Brecht, B. *Rede über die Funktion des Radios.* Gesammelte Werke, Frankfurt a.m.: Suhrkamp Verlag, 1967, Band 8.
Casey, R. H. Video Taping: A Medium for Social Change. *Instructional Technology Report.* Washington, D.C., ICIT, Academy for Educational Development, March 1974.
Elliott, P. Mass Communication—A Contradiction in Terms? In Denis McQuail (ed.), *Sociology of Mass Communications.* Middlesex, England: Penguin Books, 1972, 237-258.
Enzesberger, H. M. Constituents of a Theory of the Media. In *Sociology of Mass Communications.* op cit. 99-116.
Heap, K. *Process and Action in Work with Groups: The Preconditions for Treatment and Growth.* New York: Pergamon Press, 1979.
Ingle, H. *Communication Media and Technology: A Look at Their Role in Non-Formal Education Programs.* Information Bulletin Number Five, Washington D.C.: The Clearinghouse on Development Communication, Academy for Educational Development, August 1974.
Kalba, K. The Video Implosion: Models for Reinventing Television. In Richard Adler and Walter S. Baer (eds.), *The Electronic Box Office.* New York: Praeger, 1979.
Katz, E. and Wedell, G. *Broadcasting in the Third World.* Cambridge, Mass: Harvard University Press, 1977.
Kennedy, T. The Skyriver Project: The Story of a Process. *Challenge for Change - Access.* Montreal, National Film Board of Canada, Summer 1973, 3-21.
Lang, N. A Comparative Examination of Therapeutic Uses of Groups in Social Work and in Adjacent Human Service Professions. a) Part I - The literature from 1955-1968, *Social Work with Groups,* 1979, 2(2), 101-116. b) Part II - The literature from 1969-1978, op. cit. 1979, 2(3), 197-220.
Mallinson, T. J. Application of Group Processes to a Clinical Setting. *International Journal of Social Psychiatry,* 1965, 2, 32-37.

Mott, C. 3/4'' Video or 16 mm. Film? *Development Communication Report*, 1979, *25*, 3.

Pattison, E. M. Evaluation Studies of Group Psychotherapy. *International Journal of Group Psychiatry*, 1965, *15*, 382-397.

Picardo, M. *Il Cinema Fatto dai Bambini.* Roma: Reunti, 1974.

Rhodes Center. *Unpublished Progress Reports*, Saigon, January-June 1970.

Rosenthal, W. Social Work Group Theory. *Social Work*, 1973, *18*, 60-66.

Rosler, M. To Argue for a Video of Representation: To Argue for a Video Against the Mythology of Everyday Life. *VED*, 1979, unpaged.

Schultz, P. Communication and Social Change: *Videotape Recording as a Tool for Development* (Unpublished Report), Rome, FAO, 1974.

Shinar, D. Teleclubs in Israel. In Kalman Yaron (ed.), *Lifelong Education in Israel.* Jerusalem, Council for Adult Education, Ministry of Education and Culture, 1972, 61-71.

Stuart, M. Videotape as a Development Tool. *Issues in Communications*, London: International Institute of Communications, 1977, no. 1, 20-26.

Tannenbaum, J. A. Set for Change. *TV's Impact on Society.* Washington, D.C.: United States Information Service, 1976, 11-13.

Thenot, J. P. and Manant, J. Intervention Video a Botmeur, 1976. *VED*, (Video Exchange Directory), 1979, d-23.

Tropp, E. Social Group Work: The Developmental Approach. In J. B. Turner (ed.), *Encyclopedia of Social Work*, 1977, 17, vol. 2, New York: NASW, 1321-1328.

Tuckman, B. Developmental Sequence in Small Groups. *Psychological Bulletin*, 1965, *63*, 384-399.

VED (*Video Exchange Directory*), 1979, Vancouver, Canada, Satellite Video Exchange Society, 1979.

Vincelli, E. *Il Cinema Capovolto,* Rimini-Florence, Guaroaldi Editore, 1975.

Willener, A. *Videology and Utopia: Explorations in a New Medium,* London: Routledge & Kegan Paul, 1976.

The Jam Session:
A Study of Spontaneous Group Process

Penny Katz
Sanna Longden

ABSTRACT. This experiment describes a spontaneous jazz performance and shows that the jam session can be a useful tool for study-
ing small groups. To determine why and how it works, the author
brought together five jazz musicians and gave them three musical
tasks. They also participated in a post-performance discussion and
filled out a questionnaire to elicit their feelings about the workings of
a jam session. The jam session may be a unique group because of the
speed with which it coalesces and its use of nonverbal communication, but it also exhibits classic characteristics of small group
sociology by conforming to several basic small-group models and
principles.

While listening to a jam session whose participants were professional jazz musicians, I realized that I was watching a small group in
action, one that might have interesting implications for the study of
small group process.

On first inspection, the jam session appears to be a unique con-
figuration. It is a haphazard, unrehearsed, spur-of-the-moment ag-
gregation of musicians who inevitably achieve success by playing
spontaneously and skillfully—sometimes even masterfully—without
having the history of a well-seasoned band. Group members may be
diverse in age, sex, race, value systems, life-styles, educational
levels, and musical training; they may not even speak the same
language. Nonetheless, this group manages to be metamorphosed
from an undifferentiated entity into a solid unity capable of
sophisticated performance, using a form of communication which is

Penny Katz is a social worker at Michael Reese Hospital, 29th and Ellis, Chicago, Illinois
60616. Sanna Longden is a freelance writer in the Chicago area. The author wishes to
acknowledge her gratitude to Elaine Finnegan, MSW and lecturer at Loyola University's
School of Social Work, Chicago, Illinois, for her inspiration and suggestions throughout this
project.

largely nonverbal. Few other types of groups can operate successfully in this manner. How and why does this phenomenon work?

To find out what small group sociology can learn from the workings of a jam session, I designed and carried out an experiment, supported by my dual backgrounds as social worker and jazz aficionado. The results lead me to suggest that although the jam session is unique in some ways, it also exhibits basic characteristics of small groups.

THE EXPERIMENT

The experiment was limited in scope to duplicating the jam session atmosphere, recording the performance, and eliciting the responses of each of the musicians as to how and why it works. To accomplish these goals, certain objectives were designed, most of which were achieved despite the problems created by personal time conflicts, location selection, and lack of finances.

The first step was to gather musicians who met the following criteria: (1) racial, sexual, and age diversity; (2) no member typically a leader; (3) unacquainted with one another; and (4) highly competent improvisational instrumentalists. A group was assembled consisting of Kenny—white, early 50s, tenor saxophone and flute; Ed—white, middle 30s, tenor saxophone; Milton—black, late 20s, bass fiddle; Gloria—black, early 40s, piano; and Danny—white, late 30s, percussion. None of the five had played together before. In fact, several met for the first time 15 minutes before the jam session began, although most had known of one another through professional channels. The director of video studies at a local university arranged for the use of the school's television studio and equipment, acted as technical director, and provided camera operators and engineers.

The experiment was not without its obstacles. One of the video cameras broke the day before the taping, so a portable unit had to be pressed into service. Most of the technical personnel were amateurs and, because of the nature of the experiment, had no opportunity to rehearse. The piano supplied by the university's music department was more than a half-tone flat so the saxophone players never could adjust their instruments to play in tune. Nonetheless, jazz musicians are a hardy lot, used to adversity, and all in all the effort was remarkably successful.

The format of the musical portion of the experiment was relatively simple. The group was presented with three tasks. The first was to choose one of five swing tunes, which I named for them, and immediately play it. The second was to choose one of five predetermined ballads, or slower songs, and immediately play it. The tune choices were part of the standard repertoire of jazz musicians; there was no sheet music available. The final task was to perform a piece of sheet music containing only a sequence of chords; there was no melody and no rhythm suggestion. This chord sequence, created especially for this experiment by a local jazz musician, was harmonious but not patterned after any song which would be familiar to the performers. In this task, the musicians had to create everything but the chords and had two minutes to discuss how to do it before performing.

After the performance, I initiated a brief conversation about how they found the experience and how they explained what happens during a jam session. Then I asked them to respond in writing to a prepared questionnaire. Unfortunately, without access to the video tape, readers of this paper will not be able to enjoy the musical results of the experiment, which were clearly a success. Observers agreed that the performance was very high calibre. The interaction of the group, which is the subject here, was equally fascinating and more easily set down in words.

The Performance

On the first task of choosing one of the swing tunes, Kenny suggests, "Green Dolphin Street" and the others agree. With almost no words or pause, the bassist strums a phrase and everyone comes in as though they have been rehearsing regularly. Without any visible clues, each horn takes a solo, then the piano, bass, and drums in the traditional sequence. The musicians do not make eye contact throughout the selection, yet they seem to know instinctively when each solo is ending. It is clear as the performance progresses that the group is becoming cohesive very quickly. In the beginning, they play a little tentatively, assessing one another's contributions. Very soon, however, there is a feeling of laying back, of knowing everything is going to be fine. Several faces relax into smiles.

On the second task, after I list the ballads, there is a short pause, then Ed says, "All of them are good." "Want to do a medley?" Milton asks and there is immediate agreement. After a quick discussion of the order of tunes and keys, Milton begins a long solo on "Willow, Weep for Me" with no accompaniment. Then Danny picks it up on drums, and Gloria joins in on piano, softly at first, then with increasing dynamics. When asked later how she knew when to come in, she responded, "I just felt like it."

Out of Gloria's accompaniment comes her solo on "Lover Man," with the bass and drums quietly backing her up as she gets into it, head down, swaying. The horns, who have been standing and listening, confer in an undertone: "You want to go?" "No, you go ahead." Ken swings into "Misty," a long, soulful solo which ends exactly as Ed takes over with "What's New?" Ken smiles appreciatively at his colleague's performance. After a vigorous solo with a beautiful blending of sounds in the background, all the musicians collaborate in bringing the medley to an end. As they disengage from the music, there is pleased laughter.

As task three, the series of chords, is explained, the musicians are amused and intrigued. Milton suggests the tempo: "Let's take it down like a bossa and then swing it." He explains further, "We'll take one chorus together, we'll all play a bossa, and then you come up with a line and somebody understate it."

"Who's got the melody?" Kenny asks to general laughter.

"I think you do, Ken," says Ed, passing the buck.

"Okay," says Kenny, picking up his flute. Then he pauses—the whole melody is up to him. "Well, I don't know," he says doubtfully. "Let's do it together. But where's the bossa?"

Milton begins counting softly, "One, two, one-two-three-four," and miraculously they all begin playing, the flute singing a free-form melody above the insistent bossa nova rhythm beat out on drum and bass. The designated chords are apparently Gloria's responsibility; she puts on her glasses to read them. Ed plays the first solo chorus; Danny wags his head and closes his eyes as he strokes his cymbals. As Ed fades out, Gloria picks up the lead. When she plants a final finger at the end of a cadence, Milton begins, playing a melodic line over the accompaniment of some sparse chords from the piano. The drummer takes his solo, then the horns begin fragments of melody which alternate with the drumming. They seem completely attuned when to pick up from each other. Each group member is playing different lines which change, reform, and interlock. They feel for the finale, draw out their various notes, and bring the whole event to a satisfying conclusion. There is an unidentified sigh of relief, then laughter, a little talk, but the musicians are still not looking at one another; by now, they are facing their audience.

Post-Performance Conversation

The degree to which each of these five individuals felt as members of a group was clearly demonstrated in the post-performance conversation. When I asked Milton to explain what appeared to be some confusion as to the timing in the third selection, he accepted the responsibility by declaring that it was *his* mistake. Kenny quickly reminded us that no agreement had been reached within the group as to the timing. I asked if the last tune was harder to play than the others. Kenny said, "Not after the first two chords," and the others agreed.

When discussing how they made decisions without a designated leader, Kenny's comment was "We just sort of fell in." Gloria added, "When I'm playing with a group, I enjoy hearing what he's saying and putting something in under that, and hearing what someone else is saying. Each of us gets a chance to say something different."

I asked if it is always the soloist's decision to know when to stop. Everyone began to answer, but Gloria raised her voice as she stated, "You gotta know when a person is windin' down. Usually soloists start, and they build and build, and everyone in the band can sense when the horn player is beginning to come off his solo. He may end his solo on a phrase that catches my interest and I will start mine." The others agreed it is usually the soloist's decision. But Milton added that when he started to work professionally, the older musicians would break in and end his solo, effectively saying, "Okay, young guy, you said everything you had to say."

The question that is most difficult to answer is how the performers successfully intuit the boundaries of time, space, and dynamics to maintain the delicate balance required for a cohesive jazz group performance. "It's compatibility," Milton said. "Like common goals, common objectives. When you play music, no external stuff is happening." "I think everybody is focused," Gloria said. "You can take several different sets of the same instrumentation and get several different sounds," said Kenny, "but you'd still have the same compatibility, assuming they all had a common interest."

The group members agreed that the first two tasks were easier because they knew the songs. As Gloria said, "Everybody plays those tunes." However, they also agreed that the last task was more fun because of the challenge involved. "You got any others like that?" Gloria asked. The group ended up agreeing with Danny that they were remarkably compatible and would like to see more of one another. When asked if they'd like to do it again, there was an unhesitating chorus of "Sure, love to!"

The Questionnaire

I then handed out the questionnaire I had prepared (see appendix), which they took home and returned the following week. They all said that this task was difficult and frustrating. Through the questionnaire, I tried to discover what made the jam session such a phenomenon.

DISCUSSION

From observation of the group's interaction during the performance as well as the conversation afterwards and the questionnaire responses, I learned that a jam session demonstrates a uniqueness and an adherence to small group principles.

Jam Session as Unique

It was interesting to observe how these five individuals developed into a cohesive group in an extremely short time. This is partly because, as Ed wrote, "There are unwritten directions which have been established by tradition." The swift cohesion of this group was accelerated by an immediate acceptance of these unwritten directions. Perhaps how quickly a group unifies depends upon how long it takes to define and accept such ground rules. Other groups may not be as well-defined or as quick to consolidate because they are not as aware of such basic directions or they cannot accept them as easily. .

Jazz group ground rules were operating during this experiment. For example, it is not unusual that on the first selection, the choice of tune and tempo was made by one of the saxophonists; horn players are typically group leaders in a jazz band. However, atypically, Milton, the bass player, emerged as a strong leader on the second and third tasks. In the discussion later, he explained that the bass fiddle, formerly confined to the background, has steadily moved to the forefront and taken its place as a solo instrument. It was Milton who suggested that a medley of four ballads be played instead of one, and it was he, breaking traditional format, who took the first solo. Milton also established the rhythmic structure and tempo in the final selection.

Another ground rule is that when the musicians in a group agree on a selection, they all know the time signature, the number of musical measures in one complete chorus, and the chordal structure. All members also know that the solo format, which is almost invariably used, is the playing of an ensemble melody chorus followed by individual solos and concluded by another ensemble chorus. Usually the horn players solo first, followed by the piano, the bass, and finally the drums. This format was used in the first and third selections. Common knowledge of these ground rules gives the musicians a structure within which to work.

This particular group also worked well together because each of the musicians is a highly talented performer and each respects the others' talents. In addition, they all studied music at the college level and they all play professionally. Moreover, these people were highly motivated, by their own admission, to achieve a solid and creative group objective.

The uniqueness of the jazz group is partly based on the speed with which very separate individuals become a cohesive group and achieve the goal of making music together. In addition, it does this almost completely nonverbally. However, the musicians *are* speaking on another level and in a language they all understand. Gloria, when discussing solos, said "each of us gets a chance to say something different," and Milton wrote that he ends his solo when "he says all he needs to say." Kenny wrote he'll continue his solo "if he feels he is saying something special," and both Ed and Milton mentioned the need "to express my feelings and ideas" through jazz.

The musicians feel that playing in a spontaneous jazz group is a unique experience because of the combination of performance and creativity. Gloria wrote "I am able to experience the joy of playing with the added joy of 'creating' music, which I will never play exactly the same way again." Ed said that this is one of the few situations "where the player is the creator as well as the performer. People could take years to write a symphony and miss the direct truth

that sometimes comes about when a person is creating spontaneously.''

Perhaps the jam session concept is unique because the experience
is not repeatable. Very few human interactions can ever be
duplicated exactly, but each time the players come together, they
deliberately try to create new expressions of music. One of the main
goals of this type of group is to make a unique contribution. No one
who has heard the video tape of this experiment would be able to say
he or she had heard those old standards played before in just that
way. As Kenny said, "Each situation is special, never to be
repeated in the same way. Musicians never have the same feelings
twice. Once the statement is made, it's gone.''

Jam Session as Example of Basic Principles

In spite of its singularity, the jam session concept also conforms
to several principles of small group sociology. It demonstrates two
basic small group models, the structural-functional and the
cybernetic-growth models. (All of the following quotes are taken
from Mills, 1967, pp. 17-128.) Mills describes the structural-
functional model, which is based on work by Parsons, Bales, and
Shils, as:

. . . a goal-seeking, boundary-maintaining system whose survival is problematical. It is a mutable and transitory arrange-
ment of actions, norms, ideas, and techniques devised (though
seldom entirely consciously) to meet the demands of personal,
social, and environmental realities. It is subject not only to
constant change, but to a cessation of functions or even disin-
tegration unless real demands are adequately met. At each moment the group (through its agents) must exercise intelligence
and ingenuity, mobilize its resources, and act positively in
meeting changing demands. (p. 17)

The structural-functional model assumes "that members will be
gratified as the group progresses towards its goal" (p. 17). Certainly, the jam session fits that standard. According to Mills, the
structural-functional model makes two important contributions to
the sociology of small groups. "First, it acknowledges the role of
learning and, consequently, the role of culture and its accumula-
tion" (p. 18). It was obvious during the performance that these peo-

ple were learning from one another and each one's new knowledge increased the expertise of the group. Gloria wrote that among her personal goals in playing jazz are "exchanging ideas" and "learning new ways to play tunes," and Milton mentioned the "creative interplay" within a group setting.

The second contribution of this model is to "connect motivation of the individual member to group survival. The group must gratify its members; it must attract and sustain their interest; it must fulfill, or hold a promise of fulfilling certain of their needs" (p. 18). The needs of the five musicians who participated in this experiment were expressed in their responses to the question which asked them to list three personal goals for playing jazz in a group and then judge, on a scale of 1 (not at all true) to 5 (completely true) whether playing in this group fulfilled these goals. Fourteen of the 15 responses were a 4 or 5, showing that this group did "gratify its members."

Mills' discussion of this second contribution goes on to say: "Promise of gratification ties the member to the group and the members' investment in the group provides it with motivational energy" (p. 18). In support of this, Gloria wrote, "I believe that an 'energy field' is created when musicians come together, even for the first time. I further believe that the musicians become 'tuned' to this and spontaneous music results." Ed also talked about "the energy and creativity of the group."

The jam session also conforms to the cybernetic-growth model. Originated by Deutsch, this model

> . . . assumes the existence of group agents who observe, assess the situation, and act with consequence upon the situation they observe. When, in the face of either internal or external demands these operations are unsatisfactory or inadequate, the group suffers impairment at the least, and in the extreme, destruction. On the other hand, when conditions are favorable and the operations are effective, the group not only survives but becomes capable of monitoring itself, altering its direction, determining its own history and learning how to learn to determine its history—with the consequence that it accumulates and expands its capabilities, or *grows.* (p. 19)

Mills explains that this growth depends upon feedback. Feedback is a basic aspect of the jam session structure. Several of the musicians mentioned it on their questionnaires. Kenny said his goals are "to be stimulated by the other players, to play well enough to stimulate the others, and for us all to stimulate the listeners." Milton mentioned the "creative feedback that can't be obtained while playing alone." The growth that depends on this feedback is "not an increase in membership but an increase in capabilities for meeting a wider range of possible demands" (p. 20). Mills' description of growing groups sounds like the definition of a jam session.

> Growing groups are increasingly receptive to new signals, new possibilities, new responsibilities; they are increasingly confident both in admitting strangers and in spawning new groups; and they cross the boundaries of space and time by putting their experience in communicable form for others. From the viewpoint of the cybernetic-growth model of Deutsch, small groups are a *source* of experience, learning, and capabilities, rather than just recipients. (p. 21)

Mills adds a point which ties the jam session even more securely to the cybernetic-growth model: "Group growth . . . depends directly upon members who are both capable of personal growth, and committed to group development. . . . All information processes we have attributed to the group are actually performed by and through individuals as essential components of the collective system" (p. 21).

The members of our jazz group, when asked how a jam session manages to be successful, showed in their answers that they are very aware their group is a collection of individuals working together. Danny wrote about "the willingness to participate in a group effort to create coherent music," and Milton talked about "common goals and objectives."

Mills discusses the cybernetic-growth model's two contributions to small group sociology, and once again the jam session meets these qualifications. (1) *Its focus on momentary activity.* It "directs the outside observer's attention to the concrete moment of action . . . an important step in a theoretical model because it is precisely the realities of the concrete moment of action that confront the member of the group and that must be managed by him. . . . What the member learns about his group is relevant to the sociologist and vice versa" (pp. 22, 23). (2) *Its provision for growth.* It not only demonstrates that individuals and groups learn and grow, "but it becomes a useful analytic tool when the sociologist encounters persons and groups who are interested in more than survival and immediate gratification; whose vision for the group includes new ideas, techniques, and goals; who are willing to assume responsibility for maximizing the general capabilities of the group, and who experience gratification when the group progresses toward that end'' (p. 23).

The jam session is a good example of Deutsch's third-order group, the group in pursuit of a collective goal, which is ''an idea about a desirable state of affairs for the group as a unit'' (p. 102). A jam session also demonstrates well the distinction between affective relations and goal pursuit (p. 108). In addition, it shows clearly the generative pole of group formation ''where group emotion is simultaneously diffused to the group as a whole, and mobilized around a sense of responsibility for its future. . . . Libidinal attachment is to . . . the *idea* of creating a conflict-free group which is conducive both to individual and group growth'' (p. 120). This concept is born out in Danny's statement that he enjoys playing in a group because of the ''sharing of the responsibilities for making music,'' and in Ed's words that ''the energy and creativity of the group can exceed that of the individuals.''

Another principle of small group sociology demonstrated by this particular spontaneous jazz event is the democratic type of authority relations. In democratic groups, ''*any* member may become the official head'' and this headship is transitory: ''A subordinate ascends to authority only to return to subordination. . . . Persons in positions of authority and subordination are interchangeable'' (p. 126). The musicians were asked on the questionnaire to name the leaders who emerged in each task. There was quite a variety of responses to this question, although everyone except Milton agreed that he was the leader of the third selection. He answered that ''the collective group'' was the leader on all three. Danny said ''no one'' was leader in the first two tasks, but most of the others named Kenny as the first leader, including Kenny himself. The group members were also asked to judge by the 1-to-5 system how comfortable they were with the persons named acting as leaders, and all but one person responded with 5s for all three selections; Kenny's responses were a conservative 4. Obviously, whoever were the leaders in each situation, this is democracy in action.

Peer relations within small groups are also an important subject of study and the jam session is a precise example of the collaborative type, for according to Mills, ''Among collaborators, tension is reduced by progressive movement toward a joint goal, closeness and distance being left open to their experience together'' (p. 128). Collaborators ''are committed to a common goal'' but not to ''a given degree of intimacy.'' Milton, the bassist, sums this up when he writes that the ''common objective is to play with sympathy to the other guy.''

CONCLUSION

Based on this experiment and years of observing other spontaneous jazz groups, I suggest that the jam session can be a useful tool for the study of small group processes because of its uniqueness as well as its conformance to basic principles of small group sociology. An interesting exercise for further research might be finding other small groups that share some of the special characteristics of the jam session.

The cohesion of this particular group was further demonstrated a week after the experiment when all participants, including the video team, came together at my home for a spaghetti dinner and a review of the videotape. They obviously still felt positively connected— there was hugging and a great sense of warmth as they proudly introduced their families to one another. It was clear that the nonmusicians also felt very much a part of the group. They watched the tape with excitement and amusement, and frequently complimented one another on different passages and made good-natured comments.

REFERENCE

Mills, Theodore M. *The Sociology of Small Groups.* Englewood Cliffs, N.J.: Prentice-Hall, Inc., 1967.

JAZZ GROUP QUESTIONNAIRE

Name: _____

Instrument: _____

The following questions relate to the experiment in which you just participated. Some of the questions are in the form of a statement. For those types of questions, please fill in the blank with a number from 1 to 5 with 1 signifying that the statement is at least true and 5 signifying that the statement is most true. For example, the statement "A circle is round" should receive a 5; the statement "a triangle has four sides" should receive a 1; and the statement "Human beings are female" should receive a 3, because it is approximately half-true. Other questions require you to supply the answer. Please try to be as accurate and complete as possible in supplying these answers.

Thank you very much for participating in this experiment which is attempting to shed a little light on some of the mysteries of non-verbal communication among jazz musicians.

1. I enjoy playing jazz in a group rather than alone because:

2. My personal goals in playing jazz in a group are:

    (a)

    (b)

    (c)

3. Playing with this group fulfilled goal (a)   _____

                                                      (1 to 5)

4. Playing with this group fulfilled goal (b)   _____

                                                      (1 to 5)

5. Playing with this group fulfilled goal (c)   _____

                                                      (1 to 5)

6. All of the members of this group are competent
    musicians   _____

                                                      (1 to 5)

7. I enjoyed the experience of playing with this
    group
                                            _____
                                            (1 to 5)

8. The group played well together (1st Musical
    Selection)
                                            _____
                                            (1 to 5)

9. The group swung (1st Musical Selection) _____
                                            (1 to 5)

10. The group played well together (2nd Musical
    Selection)
                                            _____
                                            (1 to 5)

11. The group swung (2nd Musical Selection) _____
                                            (1 to 5)

12. The group played well together (3rd Musical
    Selection)
                                            _____
                                            (1 to 5)

13. The group swung (3rd Musical Selection) _____
                                            (1 to 5)

For the purposes of this questionnaire, the term "leader" will mean the
member of the group who was most involved or played the greatest role in
the decision making process (such decisions as choice of selection, order
of solos, tempos, keys, etc.)

14. _____ emerged as the leader with respect
    to the first selection.

15. _____ emerged as the leader with respect
    to the second selection.

16. _____ emerged as the leader with respect
    to the third selection.

17. I was comfortable with the person named in
    question 14 acting as leader

    _____
    (1 to 5)

18. I was comfortable with the person named in
    question 15 acting as leader

    _____
    (1 to 5)

19. I was comfortable with the person named in
    question 16 acting as leader

    _____
    (1 to 5)

20. I played well on the first selection

    _____
    (1 to 5)

21. I played well on the second selection

    _____
    (1 to 5)

22. I played well on the third selection

    _____
    (1 to 5)

23. I would have preferred it if we weren't limited
    to pre-selected tunes

    _____
    (1 to 5)

24. I liked the first selection

    _____
    (1 to 5)

25. I liked the second selection

    _____
    (1 to 5)

26. I liked the third selection

    _____
    (1 to 5)

27. The choice of songs was not important

    _____
    (1 to 5)

28. It wouldn't matter to me how the group sounded
    as long as I played well

    _____
    (1 to 5)

29. It is more important to me what the other musi-
    cians feel about how the group and its members
    sound than how the audience feels   _____
                                                   (1 to 5)

30. I would like to play with this group again   _____
                                                   (1 to 5)

31. If I had the opportunity to change any of the
    personnel, I would make the following changes
    and for the following reasons:

32. I was happier with the way the group sounded
    than with the way I sounded   _____
                                                   (1 to 5)

33. I was happier with the way I sounded than with
    the way that the group sounded   _____
                                                   (1 to 5)

34. The length of my solos was determined by the following factors:

35. Playing jazz is special because:

36. Jazz musicians who have never played together before can still get
    together and spontaneously create improvised music which depends,
    in part, on the members of the group listening to and complementing
    one another. How do you account for this?

37. The following is a brief statement about my musical educational
    background:

An Educational/Supportive Group Model for Intervention with School-Age Parents and Their Children

Linda H. Kilburn

ABSTRACT. This discussion describes the special techniques and resources required to successfully develop groups for teenage pregnant women and others with infants and toddlers. Emphasis on ways to reach-out, develop commitment through supportive contacts, useful information and personal involvement are described. A combination of program and personal investment seemed necessary to attract and hold the interest of this vulnerable population.

The Scope and Nature of Teen-Pregnancy as a Problem

In the past twenty years there have been marked changes in the incidence of teenage pregnancy, the range of choices open to the pregnant teen, and the types of programs developed to meet the needs of this population. More than 1,000,000 teenagers become pregnant each year; more than 600,000 give birth.[1] While birthrates for other age groups are dropping or remaining constant, the birthrate to the youngest group of teens, i.e., those under the age of 15, has nearly doubled.[2]

A generation ago, the solution for the unwed teenager who became pregnant was to cover it up, either via a hasty marriage or

Linda H. Kilburn is a Program Development Consultant and can be reached at 45 Metacomet Rd., Waban, Mass. 02168. She is Executive Director, Hospice of the Good Shepherd, Inc., Waban, Mass. and has also spent several years as Director, Premature Parenthood Program, Mental Health Assn. of Greater Lowell, Inc., Lowell, Mass.

by shipping the girl off to a relative or "home for unwed mothers" in a distant town. Eight out of ten babies were placed for adoption.[3] Currently, 94% of teens giving birth opt to keep and raise the child. Even among those giving birth out-of-wedlock, 87% choose to keep and raise their child.[4]

It has been well documented that the teenage parent is at risk for a variety of physical, social, educational and economic reasons. Physical immaturity, poor nutrition, inadequate health care, school drop-out and the consequent lack of skills, social pressure and the lack of economic resources are only some of the factors weighing heavily against a successful parenting experience.[5,6] These problems are accentuated for the minority teen who is often cut off from resources by language and cultural barriers as well as for the male teenage parent who is too often stereotyped as the "bad guy" and ignored in service planning.

Despite the extent of the need, a major problem faces the provider attempting to develop service models for this population: teen parents are among the least likely to seek out services. Some of the major factors acting as deterrents are:

1. Lack of knowledge about existing services,
2. Poor access to services (e.g., transportation, lack of child care services for other children, etc.),
3. Inadequate economic resources (including health insurance coverage),
4. A wish to conceal the pregnancy as long as possible,
5. Fears of retribution and punishment by parents, school and welfare authorities, employers, etc.,[7]
6. Attitudes of service providers (often demeaning, critical or unresponsive to the special needs and fears of this clientele),
7. Mistrust of adults,
8. The fear of being branded a "bad parent" and consequently having one's child taken away.

The last category is probably the one which most often affects the school-age parents' willingness to seek out services after the birth of a baby, particularly if they are experiencing parenting difficulties. Knowledge of these factors is essential to understanding both a client's reason for action (or non-action) and to developing a program which is able to overcome these barriers and increase service access and utilization.

Initiating a Program for School-Age Parents

During the period from 1973 to 1978, a comprehensive program for school-age parents was developed and implemented in the Greater Lowell area of Massachusetts, under the auspices of the Mental Health Association of Greater Lowell, Inc. The key component of the service package was an educational/supportive group model.

The program was established as the result of needs documented in the "First Baby Project," a joint venture of the Dr. Harry C. Solomon Mental Health Center and the Mental Health Association, conducted in the Spring of 1973.

Although this project was primarily designed as a needs assessment, an attempt to form a group for young mothers was made as an offshoot of the program. Fourteen young mothers were interviewed, all residents of an inner city housing project. Space for the group meetings was offered in the community center of the housing project and the services of a babysitter were contracted to care for children during the meetings. The format for the group was presented as an informal one in which members could share their experiences and concerns, discuss parenting issues, and meet others sharing similar experiences. The group was co-led by a group worker well known from her experience in the housing project's teen drop-in center and an assistant assigned from the "First Baby Project" team.

Failure and Exploration of Causes

The first group series was a failure. During the entire 10 week group series, no one attended a group meeting despite the interest expressed repeatedly during preliminary and subsequent home visits. However, despite the lack of attendance, potential group members were discovered to be calling the community center for "other reasons" during meeting time. Several sent younger siblings over to the center to "check out what was happening," and three members began attending the evening drop-in center (something they had not done previously), although they avoided direct contact with the group worker involved in the pilot Mothers' Group series.

In an attempt to ascertain the reasons for group non-attendance and to determine what suggestions members might have to make future group attempts more viable, a series of follow-up home visits was conducted. Typical comments were: "The Center has too many people in it"; "I can't get out with the baby—it's too much trouble." There were concerns about the status (single mothers) of the group, fears that the ultimate motivation of the group worker was to prove them bad mothers, and consequently take their children away. Members were also threatened by fears of not knowing anyone and by the concept of an informal group setting in which they might not know what to do or say.

A Second Attempt

The failure of this first group series provides a perfect example of how inadequate attention to the deterrents to service usage can work against a service plan. Within a year of the failed group series, the program was running 15 to 20 group series per year and making an average of 90 outreach contacts per week to clients from an 8-town area. Much of the revised group model and outreach structure were derived directly from input from prospective members of the "failed" group. Eventually, groups were developed for school-age mothers, fathers and couples. At least three series per year were conducted in Spanish. In the revised model, groups met twice a week for a period of 12 weeks. The goals of the group included:

1. Increasing members' knowledge and use of existing services
2. Increasing the number and type of socially supportive contacts
3. Improving parenting skills
4. Building a more positive parental identity

With the exception of the fathers' group, each group was staffed by a team of social worker, nurse and outreach worker. The team approach eliminated problems of overdependence on or overburdening individual staff members and provided for better coverage during off-hours.

The content of the meetings changed from series to series. It was geared to the interests and needs of members as determined through preliminary interviews plus what subsequently arose during the course of the series. The format of the group was an educational/supportive one: presentations on such topics as prenatal care, labor, delivery, child development and care, welfare and tenants' rights, family planning, and coping techniques were interspersed with informal rap sessions and peer support-building. The inclusion of a nurse to provide ongoing health and child development education and the use of concrete materials, e.g., films, greatly contributed to the improvement in attendance, particularly since the group set its own priorities. The use of outside speakers had the added benefit of acquainting members with other services, providers and agencies in a relatively non-threatening setting. This, in turn, was found to increase the likelihood that clients would utilize these services in the future.

Group membership was limited to a maximum of 12 members. The average age was 17 with the range generally running from 14 to 20. At attempt to mix ages and situations was made, i.e., each group had several pregnant members, several with infants and several with toddlers. Thus the members' personal experiences covered a wider range of parenting and child development issues and provided first-hand experiences that might be of use immediately or at a later date. For example, a discussion on potty training would be less effective if presented to a group in which all of the members were pregnant with their first child. In the mixed membership format, pregnant members had the opportunity to observe and hear about the actual parenting experiences of their peers in the group. An attempt was also made to place members from similar geographical areas in the same group. Outside-of-group contact was encouraged. Because of the option to re-enroll for a second group series, each group also had several repeaters who were familiar with the program and aided getting the group off the ground.

Key Elements of the Outreach Approach

Outreach efforts began with the careful education of staff in local agencies, clinics and organizations likely to come into contact with school-age parents. These agencies were familiarized with the program's services and staff. They were then able to describe the program to the potential client. Many referrals were also made by program participants once the program was established.

After a referral was made, a staff member went to the client's home for a preliminary interview. No client was brought into a group without having had this interview. This home visit served important purposes. For staff, there was the opportunity to observe the home situation and describe the program in detail; for the client, there was a less threatening beginning on one's own "turf" and a familiarity with at least one face when coming to a group meeting.

Often several home visits were made before a client felt comfortable enough to join a group.

Transportation was provided to and from every group meeting for each client and his/her child (children), either via the program's minibus or via volunteer drivers (for group members from outlying towns). A staff member went with the bus and met the participant at the door. The staff member could then assist the participant concretely (e.g., carrying baby equipment, assisting with a toddler, etc.) as well as urge a more hesitant member to attend. As with the preliminary home visits, these outreach pick-ups also afforded the opportunity to observe the home situation and, more importantly, to answer any questions other family members might have about the group and its intentions. This was particularly important in dealing with the mothers of the school-aged parents (one half to two thirds still lived at home). The teenage mother's own mother is often the most important support figure in her life. Thus, it was imperative to involve her as a member of the "team." She would then be more likely to support her daughter's growth rather than be threatened by new child care techniques or sabotage the group by forcing her daughter to choose between these two support and knowledge sources. The outreach effort continued on the bus ride where members had the opportunity to chat, see where each other lived and "break the ice" before the meeting.

Groups were held at various community sites such as the lounge in a women's residence at the YWCA, a location favored by the participants for its out-of-the-center-of-the-city location and privacy. A fully equipped nursery (with donated equipment) was located across the hall from group meetings. Babysitters were provided during the meetings and coffee and tea were served, with many members bringing baked goods. Fathers' groups were held in the conference room of the city library.

Special Outreach Techniques

There were several other outreach techniques which made for success in involving the school-age parent:

1. The training and employment of former program members in nearly all aspects of the program. This included a 12 week, 20 hour per week training course in outreach techniques. Each

outreach worker was assigned to one group series and also worked several days a week in the community, providing information and referral, crisis intervention and other outreach services. The program member outreach workers provided accessible role models for group members, reduced threat in outreach contacts, and, in concert with the community locations (e.g., high schools, neighborhood health clinics, housing projects, etc.), increased the program's accessibility.

2. Program members were also involved as caretakers in the program's nursery and formed the bulk of the editorial board of the monthly newsletter sent to all present and past members.

3. The newsletter, itself, was an outreach tool which provided a communication link among all program members, ongoing information and education on community resources, a massive swap-and-trade program (for baby and maternity clothes, furniture, etc.), and gave members the opportunity to work together, to use their creative talents, increase their socialization and carry tasks to completion. Although group involvement was generally limited to two group series, members were free to contact the program through its outreach centers at any time and were encouraged to maintain contact with the program through its newsletter.

4. A concentrated effort was made to build a program "family network" where members could call on each other as well as staff in times of crisis, and where members could build up sufficient social supports and concrete knowledge to reduce the stresses on themselves as young, and predominantly single, parents. The culminating expression of the "family network" was the annual family reunion picnic to which all present and past members were invited. Turnouts at these gatherings averaged from between 35 and 50 parents and up to 75 children. Every year there were representatives dating back to the earliest groups, including five members of the "failed" series who subsequently enrolled in a revised group series model.

5. One other outreach tool utilized was mailings regarding upcoming events in the group. This generally increased attendance as well as anticipation of the material.

More detailed comment needs to be made regarding the use of resource materials and speakers utilized within this type of educational/supportive group model. Clearly, no matter how dynamic any film or speaker might be, the effect will be lost unless:

1. There is sufficient outreach to get clients to attend
2. Clients feel comfortable in the group
3. Trust and rapport have been established so that clients will be receptive to new and/or threatening material
4. A feedback mechanism is used to assess the material, the speakers and members' grasp of the content

The breadth of the school-age parents' needs and their immaturity in dealing with life crises necessitates great flexibility in programming. Staff found consistently that attendance and receptivity were higher when formal materials were interspersed with open "rap" sessions where the group could adapt its focus to a specific need on a specific day. Sometimes this meant cancelling a film or a speaker on a given day, even with little prior notice. Issues of importance, e.g., fears regarding an impending birth, a young parent's difficult scene with his/her own parent or child, needed to take precedence for the group to sense its ownership of the program.

A Review of Resources

Below are more specific resources utilized in the educational/supportive group format:

1. *People* (Staff, guest speakers, program member role models and the program members themselves). Clearly, the staff were the key to the initial success of the model. They performed the outreach necessary to encourage and maintain member participation. Guest speakers were helpful in bringing new perspectives and specific information plus giving clients first-hand knowledge of other providers and services. The indigenous outreach workers were also important; they were drawn from the program, trained, and served as attainable role models. They reinforced members' sense of self-worth and contributed insights into their peers' needs and concerns, making for better program planning. The program members offered each other support, helpful hints and suggestions, and reassurance of the bond of commonality among them.

2. *Specific Content and Resource Persons.* Child growth and development (child psychologists and staff members from an early

intervention program), apartment security and screening of strangers (members of the police department), tenants' rights and housing related concerns (speakers from the housing authority, code department and citizens' advocacy groups), welfare rights (speakers from the Department of Public Welfare and citizens' advocacy groups), diet and nutrition (speakers from the Department of Public Health, Visiting Nurse Association and county extension service which also had excellent films on diet and pregnancy), consumer education (speakers from the U.S. Consumer Product Safety Commission), potty training (pediatric nurse specialists and program staff), birth control and family planning (speakers from the Family Planning Clinic and program staff), emergency first aid and artificial respiration (Red Cross speakers), child care (nursing staff and visiting pediatricians), when to call the doctor and caring for children when they are sick (same as above), make-up and grooming (visiting beauticians), educational and vocational opportunities (high school and G.E.D. personnel; Department of Public Welfare; personnel from local vocational training programs), drugs, alcohol and smoking, including effects on pregnancy (program staff and personnel from local drug program), pregnancy, labor and delivery (childbirth instructors, program staff), child care operations (personnel from Head Start, pre-school and early intervention programs, local day care centers), lead paint poisoning, symptoms and treatment (speakers from Department of Public Health and local lead paint testing program), legal rights (speakers from Legal Aid Bureau, private lawyers and Department of Public Welfare), exercises for pregnancy, postnatal, dieting and general improved health (program nursing staff and personnel from YWCA), rape crisis (representative from local rape crisis center), battered women (representative from local program). With few exceptions, these outside speakers donated their time and were highly supportive of the group's efforts to bring clients into closer and more knowledgeable contact with area resources.

3. *Films, filmstrips, video-tape and cassettes.* Audio-visual aids were screened for their brevity, simplicity of presentation and appeal to younger audiences. Some examples and sources included *The Child, Human Sexuality* (Unitarian Universalist Education Department), *Self Breast Examination* (American Cancer Society), *Emergency First Aid* (Red Cross), *Newborn; The First Three Months of Life* (Association Sterling Films), *Menstruation, Birth Control* and *Venereal Disease* (Family Planning Clinic films), *Don't*

Give Up On Me (Children's Protective Service); *Born with a Habit* (Harvard Medical School), *Old Enough to Know* (Planned Parenthood League), *Teenage Father* (Planned Parenthood League), *Filmstrip Series on the Teen Parent* (Parents' Magazine), *Children in Crisis* (Parents' Magazine), *Child Development: Birth to 18 Months* (Parents' Magazine), *Child Behavior: Birth to Age 5* (Parents' Magazine), *Everyday Problems of Young Children* (Parents' Magazine), *Toy Safety* and *The Travels of Timothy Trent* (both put out by the U.S. Consumer Product Safety Commission).

4. *Printed Materials.* The materials which were found to be the most effective were those which were concise, used simple, straightforward language and were illustrated with bright photos or graphics. One extremely useful tool for reinforcing material covered in group sessions was the provision of a resource folder. This manila envelope was given to each member at the beginning of the series and was utilized for keeping materials given out in meetings. Initially, the only items in the folder were a list of group members' names, addresses, phone numbers, children's names and ages (or due dates!) and staff numbers (office and emergency). Added into the folders during the course of the series were such items as an emergency phone number card, a poison antidote chart and poison center phone number, community clinic schedules, pamphlets given out by speakers, printed hand-outs designed by staff for group meetings, and a simple, four page mini-resource directory of services in the area likely to be utilized or needed by program participants. Other printed resource materials included the program's monthly newsletters, printed in English and in Spanish.

Conclusion

The key to the success of the educational/supportive group model lay in the basic principles of outreach and networking. Provision of transportation (a *must* even if the program is located in one neighborhood), babysitting, inclusion of program members in all aspects of the program, extensive home visiting, location of the program site in a non-threatening and private setting, staff team approach, use of the newsletter and mailings as a communication link, involvement of the family or significant other in the program, and lastly, the concentrated effort to build a family network, met with success in getting the often mistrustful teen to services where they could build self-sufficiency and improve their parenting skills. The success of the intervention was born out in formal evaluation of 27 of the group series conducted over a four year period. Member responses to pre- and post-group series interview/questionnaires indicated statistically significant (at the .005 level) improvement in their knowledge and use of existing services within the community, number and type of socially supportive contacts, and feelings of competence in caring for their children. In addition, parental attitude studies conducted within the interview/questionnaire format, provided important insights for staff into the intergenerational family dynamics and role-modeling sources for the school-age parents participating in the program.[8]

NOTES

1. Alan Guttmacher Institute. *11 Million Teenagers,* Planned Parenthood Federation of America, Inc., New York: 1976 (p. 10).

2. Boston Hospital for Women Division of Affiliated Hospitals Center, Inc. "For Your Information Fact Sheet," Boston: 1978.

3. Sauber, Mignon and Corrigan, Eileen M. *The Six Year Experience of Unwed Mothers as Parents,* Community Council of New York, New York: 1970 (p. v).

4. Alan Guttmacher Institute. *11 Million Teenagers,* p. 11.

5. Steinmetz, Pearl, and Teele, James, Editors. *The Unwed Mother, Issues in Preventive and Helping Services,* Boston: United Community Services of Metropolitan Boston, 1974 (p. i).

6. Osofsky, Howard J., M.D. *The Pregnant Teenager, A Medical, Educational and Social Analysis,* Springfield, Illinois: Charles Thomas Publisher, 1968 (pp. 21-28).

7. *Ibid.,* pp. 27-28.

8. Kiser, Linda Kilburn. "An Educational/Supportive Group Experience in Work with School-Age Parents and Their Children," graduate thesis available in the Mugar Library of Boston University, Boston, Mass.

Poetry Writing Groups
and the Elderly:
A Reconsideration of Art
and Social Group Work

George S. Getzel

ABSTRACT. The historical relationship between the arts and social group work is examined through work done in poetry writing groups of the elderly. The skills used in these groups are delineated and examples of poetry are analyzed. The intrinsic value of the elderly's poetry is emphasized over an instrumental view of arts as media.

Poetry writing in groups with the elderly and the handicapped is an idea that quickly stirs interest and excitement. Social workers, poets, recreational therapists, nurses, psychiatrists and amateurs have begun to test out the approach. This paper will examine poetry as art in the practice of social group work. A good many of the insights presented are derived from the Artists and Elders Project directed by Marc Kaminsky, a program which trained poets and social workers to work with groups of the elderly in senior citizen centers, nursing homes and rehabilitation settings in New York City under grants from C.E.T.A. and a private foundation.

For a social group worker, poetry writing has a familiar ring. It seems to be another type of program media that may help people. What makes it special or unique? How does it influence the process or direction of social group work practice? The characteristics of

George S. Getzel is an Associate Professor, Hunter College School of Social Work of the City University of New York, 129 East 79th St., New York, N.Y. 10021.

poetry, poetry writing and group development will be identified from the practitioner's perspective. A major emphasis will be upon the historical relationship between the arts and practice, and possible new directions suggested by the widespread experimentation with poetry writing groups.

THE ARTS AND SOCIAL GROUP WORK

The arts and social work with groups have had a long and continuous association. In the late part of the 19th century, the social settlement movement identified popular participation in the arts as an important goal. Jane Addams (1910) described Hull House residents in their endeavors of exposing great literature to bewildered immigrant youngsters. Romantic Victorian thinking endowed the arts with the power to instill cultivated and humane values in the poor and the disadvantaged.

Lillian Wald (1934) of the Henry Street Settlement underlined the importance of the informal presentation of educational and cultural experiences in club groups and non-graded classes. She saw the arts as an antidote to the Puritan heritage which she felt inhibited the expression of "play and joy and beauty." Miss Wald wrote:

> Through the informal workshops and studios, through recreation as well as through the beautiful festivals and the plays, through music and opportunities that have presented themselves, intertwining education and the arts, it is impressed upon us that the world has barely awakened to the force and importance that may be afforded to old and young, to the happy, to the weary and to the inhibited. (164, 174)

In 1922, Woods and Kennedy (1922) who surveyed social settlements pointed out that the initial emphasis on exposing neighborhood people to great art was gradually replaced by the engagement of the people themselves in producing their own art and sharing it with others in the community. Exhibitions of folk art, for example, were seen as ways of generating understanding and amity among different ethnic populations. The art itself might provide employment and income for artists and artisans. Musical, visual and dramatic arts were generally used in settlement houses. The arts were to be "understood, honored and conserved" even in the poorest neighborhood, because they were necessary for the common education of new Americans and ultimately for the refinement of the individual.

The arts as planned program activities in small groups became an essential component of the early efforts to formalize and define social group work practice. These activities were believed to be intrinsically enhancing to the individual who was denied an outlet for self-realization. Moreover, the arts provided a basis for group acceptance and socialization, and had the potential of contributing to social solidarity. The arts, in short, were seen as a broad means to personal and social ends. Art as an end in itself with its own inherent purpose was not a strong emphasis.

For the most part, theorists and scaffolders of social group work practice see the arts as categories of *instrumental* activities with less attention to the product of the activities. Wilson and Ryland (1949) write:

> Each activity has peculiar qualities which appeal to certain individuals and are important factors in the choice as program. But its values need not be peculiar to the activity; many of the same values can result from activities, which on the surface, seem to be very different. (p. 153)

Instrumentalism turns the arts into activities closely allied to informal education and recreation. In part this may be explained by early groups workers' attention to the needs of children and adolescents. Grace Coyle (1947) in her classical statement of the function of program activity sees it as a means to enhance satisfaction in human relations, to help people incapable of enjoying themselves find satisfaction through others and to contribute to members' health, education and participation in the broader society. More recently Middleman (1968) has expressed a similar view that "program is the vehicle through which relationships are made and the needs and interests of the group and its individuals are fulfilled" (p. 67).

Helen Phillips (1957) views activity as offering opportunities for the creation of experiences and group products that must be understood in their own right. Groups can and do make their own unique creative forms that were heretofore unknown to the worker and group members.

There is no mechanical way of describing group process as it evolves around activities or issues or ideas, for it develops as people relate to each other and is creative only as its participants find expression for their real selves and are free to take in, and respond to, the real feelings and ideas of others. (p. 146)

Experience with poetry writing groups supports Phillips' notion. While this activity may benefit individuals, the product cannot be divorced from the process. The product or the poetry has a special meaning for the elderly and people from other generations who read it. The group process is an intimate reflection of the poetry created.

PREPARATION

As a social worker plans to engage a group of the elderly in poetry writing, he has doubts about his ability to succeed. The worker faces a powerful dilemma between his belief in the natural drive that all people have to create something outside themselves and his perceptions of the bodily decline and societal stigma the aged bear. The generative synthesizing aspect of art seems to be contradicted by human aging associated with faltering steps and waning powers. Experience with these groups has taught us not to deny our doubts and our feelings but to see them as reflections of the thoughts old people may be experiencing. It is important to allow tentativeness, fears and ambivalence to be expressed in the group and in the poetry.

PRACTICE PHILOSOPHY

Butler and Lewis (1974) describe loss as the predominate emotional theme of aging. Losses of spouse, friends, health, social status and economic security are likely occurrences for many older persons. How do you "work through," "adapt" or "cope" to losses of people or situations which have conventionally defined your personhood? In fact, mental health concepts sound hollow and false as responses to the losses of old age.

We see poetry as creative expressions of the developmental strivings of old people to handle loss and to redefine themselves at a richer, more complex level. The pain from losses is not necessarily soothed but; by writing poetry, it may be heroically encountered.

Powerful themes seem to undergird the poetry of old people. First, they wish to make a statement that their existences are not wholly contingent on the past and its symbols of success. Despite possible failures as parents, spouses, friends and workers, they still want to believe in their intrinsic worth in the face of self-doubt and the indifference of others. Second, they seek a vision of themselves which transmutes the bodily wounds and the hurts of aging, and speaks of an enduring personality savoring the past and the present. Third, they grapple with the meaning of living in the face of personal death. The poem is a touchstone of remembrance, something old people leave behind for others to read. Writing a poem is inextricably tied to an encounter with the boundaries of time that surround every human life.

Rollo May (1975) tells us being human is defined by the creative life:

> The essence of being human is that, in the brief moment we exist on this spinning planet, we can love some people and some things, in spite of the fact that time and death will ultimately claim us all and that we yearn to stretch the brief moment to postpone our death. (p. 19)

The elderly in writing groups learn about each other's efforts to leave behind tracings of their past, visions of a world they created and a world that remains for others to create. Through their poems they share a legacy with the worker and with their children, grandchildren and unknown future generations.

The centrality of transmitting permanent statements of old people's generational experiences underlies group members' behavior. Old people in groups are creating contemporary epic poems linking them to the past and the future.

Poetry writing is defined as work because it produces a permanent product. Like all work, it always betrays its human hallmark. In the beginning of the group, old people work on two interrelated tasks. The first is to determine the kind of group they want and the second to make poetry. Group ties and norms do not come easily. Nonetheless, when poetry and group interaction happen together, enhanced stimulation and reinforcement of purpose are possible.

PHASES OF GROUP DEVELOPMENT

Four phases tend to occur in poetry writing groups which are related to the obstacles found in the group over time. The following are statements of the worker's focus and descriptions of each phase.

Phase 1: The worker opens up the theme of the members' distrust of their creative abilities

In the beginning of the group, participants doubt they can write poetry. Their distrust of themselves may be so intense and pervasive that it appears tightly encoded in their non-verbal behavior. The worker openly shares his belief in their abilities. Frequently, old people doubt their creativity because previous occupations afforded them few opportunities for artistic expression. They distrust those who view them as capable. In the beginning phase of the group, the worker carefully structures opportunities for group members' first poetic attempts. The use of group or shared poems is very effective. Each member contributes a line of poetry on a theme suggested by the group or the worker. Themes such as dreams, holiday, water, and food permit the sharing of thoughts and poetic ideas in a considered manner, while members listen to one another.

For example, the worker and the group may talk about how it feels to be old. They come upon the theme of "getting old." The worker suggests that members close their eyes and see their own pictures of "getting old." Each offers a line of poetry.

Getting Old

(A) Gray dandelion seeds rising in the air
(B) A dry twig breaking,
(C) I sit alone in the house waiting for my son,
(D) Don't be sad, spring is coming,
(E) It isn't so bad.

The poem is an individual and collective expression of feelings and associations that creates a statement giving form to otherwise inchoate ideas. Participants A and B make use of similar natural images, at once challenging and subtly reinforcing the other. C's images mirror B's sad tone. D comforts A, B and C as E abruptly

brings closure to the effort by a self-referential, concrete association. Taken together the poem is a richly textured creation reflecting
members' ambivalence and shared strivings.

The group worker must be aware of his style of relating to
members. Kenneth Koch (1977), in his writing workshops with the
impaired elderly in nursing homes, states that the worker should
support members by focusing on the words they write rather than
their personal characteristics. By responding to poems, the group
worker is treating members as adults. To do otherwise is to confirm
subtly the societal stereotypes which contribute to the aged person's
depression and sense of helplessness.

The worker listens carefully for signs of appreciation as poetry is
shared. He lends his energy and enthusiasm by exploring the mean-
ings of images and ideas embedded in their works. The worker risks
the examination of the positive and the negative reactions among
group members during this phase.

Phase 2: The worker explores themes of hopelessness in the poems and in the group interaction

As group members become productive creators, they begin to
respond to the underlying themes of hopelessness—opportunities
missed, declining physical abilities, and the loss of friends and
relatives. Behind group members' avoidance and shadow boxing
behaviors is the question: "Can I still see myself as a whole enduring human being, still facing life's challenges despite the ravages of
disease and painful losses?" The group with the assistance of the
group worker slowly acknowledges these feelings.

Phase 3: The worker explicitly accepts the validity of pain and tragedy in their poetry and in their statements in the group

Enhanced intimacy among group members supports open and
sustained discussion of the fears and the effects of aging. The
worker may become a symbol of what the elderly have lost. They
may direct their anger towards him. The worker must be prepared
to hear their detailed stories filled with pain, illness, and death. By
carefully attending to group members' somber reflections, the
worker demonstrates his belief that they can face the demands of aging. The group becomes lively as poetry serves as a cathartic outlet.

Poetry, the healer, was a theme introduced by worker, Rochelle

Ratner (1980), in an Artists and Elder group in a rehabilitation center. A woman wrote her own psalm directed to God or Fate.

Heal Body Heal

What have I done to you to justify
What you have done to me, all unknowingly?
Tell me, can you heal as well as destroy,
If so, how?
If so, tell me — I shall do
As you say.

At a later time in the group Ratner asked group members to respond to the part of their body that does not work. A woman in the group wrote the following excerpt:

Right hand,
Why do you fail me?
I always took care
of you,
Kept you warm
as I could in winter,
even if
I had to sit on you.
Sorry if it hurts more
When you were cold.
At least I tried,
Why don't you
Try harder
you can do it,
I know you can
So let's keep going, trying,
Together.

Writing poems makes group members think of themselves in terms of others. Together they explicitly address the submerged questions: What should I do in the time remaining? What does it mean to live and to live this long? Reminiscence in poetry is evidence of the active use of the past to handle the problems of today. The group provides an arena for the questions of ultimate meaning.

Marc Kaminsky (1974), a poet and a social worker who has pioneered the use of poetry with the elderly, writes that the worker "Is not afraid of identifying with persons whom society habitually shuns" (p. 89). The poetry provides an acceptable cultural form which aids the members in sharing powerful and overwhelming feelings.

In a senior center, an old lady in the Kaminsky's (1980) group wrote of nature's cycles with a personal twist (p. 20).

Span of Life

The planting of a tree, the beginning.

Time passes

And the sprouting of a small shoot

Growing, scraggly, gangly, awkward
Not knowing where it's going

Tall, straight, proud, accomplished
Wiser, all knowing where it's going

Older, stauncher, calmer, settled.

Grey, aging, bending, waning
Slowly passing to its beginning
To dust returning.

Phase 4: The worker assists the development of a culture that fosters the exploration of artistic ideas and a structure which provide maximum autonomy for the group

The worker seeks to relinquish the aura of expertise gathered during the early phases of the group, as he wrestles with his need to be needed, particularly as group members' contributions become more sophisticated. He learns to credit their growth. Attention to the poetry and the group process safeguards members' autonomy.

The group is an ever changing universe comprised of people who reveal their shifting perceptions, emotions, and expectations. The worker becomes a willing servant of their artistic needs and uses a variety of artistic structures which individuals bend to their requirements. Among the useful structures that aid the group are the keeping of journals, meditations over objects of beauty, and readings of great poetry of the past. Journals have been particularly helpful in capturing the details of daily life—its trials and simple pleasures. The works of poets in late life, Yeats and Auden, for example, are sympathetically heard by group members. Reactions to the events of the day or to dreams that kept them up at night may be a rich lode of poetic inspiration.

The voice of the past comes in a dream to a woman in a group conducted by poet Jeff Wright (1980, p. 42).

A Dream

I dreamt of a mountain high and steep.
There I was toiling up toward the top.
Then nearer the top I was stunned by fear.
Out of nowhere a man appeared,
with extended arms
He helped me up to the top.
That hand to me was that of God, because of its
gentle and kindly touch.

Then and there I vowed to serve him more.
Looking around I saw a crowd.
In that crowd was my mother who has
long gone on before, beckoning to me to follow her.
We crossed a rippling stream to a great green panorama.
Then she disappeared from view leaving me alone.
A "beautiful garden" of assorted flowers I saw there.
What an array of colors!
It seemed to so real and inviting
while other dreams I had before were so frightening.

The vagaries of life and artistic inspiration aside, the group is a sanctuary from an unpredictable and unfeeling world. Kaminsky (1974) writes:

One of the most vital things that happens in poetry groups is that several individuals discover that they are not alone in feeling as they do about parents or children or their husbands; that they are not alone in their envy; that they are not alone in their self-involvement or their sense of loss, of their generous acts; that they are not alone. (p. 89)

THE POWER OF POETRY

Poetry writing in groups as artistic expression runs counter to the conventional ways of thinking about social work practice. Both the writing process and the poetry produced are *as important* in their impact on group members. As poetry is written, it takes on its own life; it represents an individual's effort to go beyond the particular aspects of existence and to reach for universal mysteries and visions.

Poems are similar to rituals which communalize a special event and sanctify it. Poetry encourages reverie. Heightened emotions and recognitions are born anew in the reader. Poems suspend the corrosive flow of time.

The ineffable aspects of aging come alive in the work. Old people's poems are signs of indebtedness and statements of existence that cry out to be heard and to be remembered. The healing function of poetry is apparent when group members create beauty as a means of combating losses. Flights into beauty—mountains, flowers, blue lakes, cherubic grandchildren are frequent themes. Nature seems to represent a purer state of being.

Social workers exploring poetry writing in groups are identifying the artistic needs of the elderly. Social workers have begun to see the arts as a means of therapy in recent years, but not as a means to directly satisfy the creative needs of persons throughout the life cycle.

Harold Lewis (1980) identifies four ways to meet the artistic requirements of people:

1. Through the direct production of art;
2. Through observation of the artistic process and art itself;
3. Through the appreciation of aesthetically appealing environments;
4. Through experiences that are designed as a form of therapy.

Poetry writing groups, as described in this paper, correspond to the first two artistic domains. Art is not seen as directly therapeutic in these groups, but as mode of self-realization and developmental enhancement. These groups have been used with old people from varied ethnic and socioeconomic backgrounds. It is clear these groups tap the old people's profoundest concerns. Their poetry is for persons of different generations. We have much to learn by reading their poetry and listening to its messages.

Poetry, the visual arts, drama, music and dance have not been seen as especially relevant to social group workers in the last twenty years. If we deny our interest in the arts, we are missing a significant area of life for the people we serve. The art that develops in groups through our actions will have the potential of broadening altruism through explicating the pains and the joys of the people we serve. We must begin to understand artistic expression in late life among a range of people. Art has the capacity to liberate the spiritual in this age of false spirits and disappointments.

REFERENCES

Addams, J. *Twenty Years at Hull House,* New York: Macmillan, 1910, pp. 371-399.

Butler, R.N. and Lewis, M.I. *Aging and Mental Health,* Second Edition, St. Louis, C.V. Mosby Co., 1977.

Coyle, G.L. *Group Experience and Democratic Values,* New York: Woman's Press, 1947, pp.69-80.

Lewis, H. Position Statement for Hunter College School of Social Work, 1980.

Kaminsky, M. *What's Inside of You It Shines Out of You,* New York: Horizon Press, 1974.

Kaminsky, M. (Ed.) *The Journal Project: Pages From Lives of Old People,* New York: Teachers and Writers Collaborative, 1980.

Koch, K. *I Never Told Anybody,* New York: Random House, 1977.

May, R. *The Courage to Create,* New York: W. W. Norton, 1975.

Middleman, R. R., *The Non-Verbal Method in Work With Groups,* New York: Association Press, 1968.

Phillips, H. U., *The Essentials of Social Group Work Skill,* New York: Association Press, 1957.

Wald, L., *Windows on Henry Street,* Boston: Little, Brown and Co., 1934.

Wilson, G. and Ryland, G., *Social Group Work Practice,* Cambridge, Mass.: Houghton Mifflin Co., 1949, p. 153.

Woods, R. A. and Kennedy, A. J., *The Settlement Horizon,* New York: Russell Sage Foundation, 1922.

Wright, J. (Ed.), *Over the Years,* New York: Teachers and Writers Collaborative, 1980.

The Use of Photography Activities with Adolescent Groups

Nancy R. Darrow
Mary T. Lynch

ABSTRACT. This paper will discuss the use of photography and videotape in unstructured early adolescent girls' therapy groups. The focus is on two illustrative groups and explores the use of these activities in various stages of the groups' development. Adolescent issues of identity, sexuality and aggression were among the themes observed.

Introduction

Planning early adolescent activity groups can be a challenge. The materials typically available in latency age activity groups are not consistent with the developmental level and interests of this age group. However, early adolescents are often not yet at the point of being able to utilize a totally discussion-oriented group. In this paper some alternate techniques for use in adolescent groups will be explored. A particular focus will be on using photography and videotape in unstructured early adolescent girls' groups.

The two groups which will be discussed were held in the outreach office of the Worcester Youth Guidance Center which is a state and locally funded child guidance clinic in Worcester, Massachusetts. The outreach office is located in a multi-racial, multi-ethnic subsidized housing project with approximately four hundred and fifty apartment units and approximately sixteen hundred residents. A high percentage of the population are children and adolescents. The

Nancy R. Darrow and Mary T. Lynch are clinical social workers at the Worcester Youth Guidance Center, 275 Belmont St., Worcester, Mass. 01604, an outreach center in a subsidized housing project.

77

racial composition is roughly 1/3 white, 1/3 black and 1/3 Hispanic with a smaller percentage of Vietnamese and Laotians.

Launching the Groups

A prime focus in the outreach office has been on groupwork and the majority of the referrals have been obtained through outreach to the neighborhood schools. A number of early adolescent girls' groups for twelve to fourteen year old junior high school girls have been offered. The groups have had five to eight members and have been held weekly through the school year. The groups were composed of black, Hispanic and white members. Some of the girls had problems which included depression, immaturity, truancy, inappropriate aggressiveness, and overwhelming anxiety. In addition, all the members seemed to be dealing with normal adolescent concerns.

In trying to form the groups the therapists visited area schools and met with the guidance counselors. A letter from the leaders describing the group and an attached parental permission slip were left with the guidance counselors who gave these to girls who might be interested. Those who returned the permission slips were contacted by the leaders for pre-group screenings. In the screenings the girls were told about the activities which would be available for their use and were also told that they might discuss any particular concerns they might have. At this time the leaders stressed that this would be the girls' group for them to plan to do what they wished and that the leaders would not be coming in with a pre-planned agenda for them. This was explained to the girls since the leaders' orientation was to use an unstructured process-oriented approach. The group leaders, although active, were non-directive.

A variety of activities were available including photography, videotape, art, cooking and games. In this article the use of photography and videotape will be described since these were the most frequently used activities. Photography and video seemed conducive to exploring adolescent issues of identity, sexuality and aggression.

Photography and Videotape as Activities

First we will review the literature on the use of photography and videotape in groups which revealed that the major themes in the articles included the effects of their use on self-image, self-perception and observing ego (Colson, 1979; Cornelison and Arsenian, 1960; Danet, 1968, 1969; Mayadas and O'Brien, 1973; Stewart, 1979; Stoller, 1967, 1969).

The first photography was available to the public in 1839, introduced by Louis Daguerre. It was first used in treatment during the 1850s by Dr. Hugh Diamond (Stewart, 1979). He was a psychiatrist in England who saw therapeutic value in showing mental patients pictures of themselves. Videotape was first used in conjunction with therapy in 1953; at that time Tucker, Lewis, Martin and Over broadcast group therapy hours over closed circuit T.V. in a psychiatric hospital and found that patients who watched also showed improvement.

Cornelison and Arsenian (1960) studied the effects on self-image of viewing Polaroid snapshots. A group of hospitalized psychiatric patients who were shown photographs of themselves immediately after they were taken were found to be more responsive to subsequent therapy than the control group who had not been shown photographs of themselves. Several other authors describe how videotaping group therapy sessions allows for a unique method of feedback in that it permits group members to observe their own behavior as others see it (Mayadas and O'Brien, 1973; Danet, 1969). The visual impact and the responses of the other group members and the therapists can facilitate a new level of self-awareness and can at times confront a client's denial of certain aspects of his behavior (Mayadas and O'Brien, 1973). The procedure of videotaping group sessions in itself may give the members the feeling that the group has a valuable purpose (Czajkoski, 1968). In a recent article on photography, Colson stresses its function as an extension of the ego:

> The camera is an analogue of certain ego processes thereby allowing conflicts about the exercise of those functions to become externalized and subject to a greater sense of mastery and control. (Colson, 1979, p. 280)

Cameras, color film and videotape equipment were among the materials available for use in the unstructured early adolescent girls' groups. Polaroid cameras were obtained through a grant from the Polaroid Corporation. Video equipment could be obtained from the local library if the group planned on this in advance.

Group Development Stages and Camera Usage

The use of these materials by the girls in various stages of group development will be explored, focusing on the themes of closeness and issues around identity and aggression as shown in two groups. Garland, Jones, and Kolodny's model of stages of group development will be employed in looking at the groups (Garland, Jones and Kolodny in Bernstein, ed., 1965).

The idea of using cameras in a group seemed to have special appeal to the girls when they were approached during outreach in trying to form the groups. A general aura of interest and excitement and a feeling that this would be "something new" prevailed when we met the girls during screening sessions.

Over the course of both groups, similar stages in the use of the cameras were observed. Initially, the girls tended to look toward the leaders as teachers who would direct the photography. Approach-avoidance feelings seemed evident in the girls' uncertainty about whether or not they would want their pictures to be taken by other group members. A great amount of anxiety about the use of cameras was evident, in contrast to the girls' earlier excitement. They approached the cameras gingerly but hesitated about taking them out of the boxes. However, the girls wavered back and forth about whether or not they wanted to receive any instruction in the use of the cameras. Initial experimental pictures were taken randomly, without any sense of planning.

In both groups, the first planned pictures were of the group leaders. Members independently decided on this subject and asked the leaders to go outside into the housing project courtyard. They then lined up before the leaders as if we were a tourist attraction in a foreign country and snapped pictures. Only after each group had symbolically appropriated the leaders in this fashion did they move on to other subjects. The girls' first moves to other subjects were accompanied by much movement back to the group leaders. They asked us to hold their pictures, give comments, etc., as they went from taking a new picture back to touching base with the leaders.

The girls appeared to use the cameras as a vehicle to allay their anxiety and give them a sense of control over new subjects. Both groups moved in parallel stages. First they took pictures of the leaders, then snapped shots of each other. Next they moved to exploring relatively safe subjects within the housing project such as taking pictures of friends, little girls and dogs. They then asked others in the housing project for permission to take photos, and finally photographed areas of Worcester beyond the housing development.

The aggressive element referred to in the literature on photography (Sontag, 1977) inherent in the use of the camera became evident as the group progressed past the initial meetings. The girls "took" pictures of each other especially when a subject showed unwillingness to pose. During this stage one girl was observed chasing a would-be subject. Another was seen pulling on the shirt of her prey, trying to get him to face the camera. During this stage there were many power and control issues, as the girls vied for the "best" photographic subjects, such as a popular neighborhood boy, and also competed to be able to take the most pictures. At times recently developed photos were literally taken from the photographer by a disgruntled fellow member.

As the groups became more cohesive and the members became somewhat less competitive with each other, the subject of videotaping was raised by each. One group chose to use videotaping at times; the other group decided against its use for reasons which are unclear. In the group which used videotape, the first theme chosen seemed to reflect a continuation of some of the power and control issues described above, but focused more on the members' relationships with the therapists. The girls planned a skit which they wanted to videotape; they cast the group leaders as controlling schoolteachers, "Miss Crabapple and Mrs. Sourpuss" and themselves as rebellious pupils. In the skit the class ended up overthrowing the teachers and banishing them from the classroom.

Viewing the videotape ushered in a period when the group discussed more openly their feelings and concerns about themselves and each other. This also was the case in viewing their photography and other subsequent videotapes.

Both groups reached the stage of being able to plan and sustain their photographic endeavors and at this point placed increased emphasis on the quality of the finished pictures. It was during this period that the girls used their works to talk about concerns about body image and racial and sexual identity. They seemed to gain comfort in discussing these subjects both because of the intimacy of the groups and because the photography gave them a certain freedom to approach these subjects and to really look at themselves and each other. The question "How do I look?" was approached by the girls on a variety of different levels, including sexual development and ethnic heritage, hair, body, color of skin, and language spoken, as they explored differences and similarities. One group planned a videotaped dance sequence and then used this to focus on some of these issues.

In dealing with termination, both groups initially regressed to taking pictures in a fashion similar to initial meetings. They shot photos without a sense of planning or organization, not wanting to stop. After a period, however, both groups moved to using photographs already taken to review what had taken place in the group, looking back somewhat nostalgically. They also planned photos of the group as a whole similar to graduation pictures. They seemed to be using the photos both as a means of keeping the group with them and as a way of dealing with termination issues. Neither group chose to use the cameras during final sessions, but instead planned parties and talk sessions. One of the girls summed up feelings about the group: "We take pictures, and laugh, and make friends better."

Conclusion

To summarize, both adolescent girls' groups which have been discussed in this paper reflected many of the issues described in the photography and videotape therapy literature. The stages observed in the two groups were similar. Themes included adolescent conflicts about their sexual and racial identities and their aggressive feelings as well as their wishes for closeness within the group. Photography and videotape seem to offer a useful vehicle for expressing some of these conflicts and concerns which are frequently hard for adolescents to convey verbally.

REFERENCES

Berger, Milton, et al. "The Use of Videotape with Psychotherapy Groups in a Community Mental Health Service Program," *International Journal of Group Psychotherapy,* Vol. 18, pp. 504-515, 1968.

Colson, Donald B. "Photography as an Extension of the Ego," *International Review of Psycho-Analysis,* Vol. 6, pp. 273-282, 1979.

Cornelison, F. S. and Arsenian, J. A. "A Study of the Responses of Psychotic Patients to Photographic Self-Image Experience," *Psychiatric Quarterly,* Vol. 34, pp. 1-8, 1960.

Czajkoski, E. H. "The Use of Videotape Recordings to Facilitate the Group Therapy Process," *International Journal of Group Psychotherapy,* Vol. 18, pp. 516-524, 1968.

Danet, Burton. "Self Confrontation in Psychotherapy Reviewed: Videotape Playback as a Clinical and Research Tool," *American Journal of Psychotherapy,* Vol. 22, pp. 245-257, 1968.

Danet, Burton. "Videotape Playback as a Therapeutic Device in Group Psychotherapy," *International Journal of Group Psychotherapy,* pp. 440-443, 1969.

Garland, James, Jones, Hubert, and Kolodny, Ralph. "A Model for Stages of Development in Social Work Groups," in Bernstein, Saul, ed., *Explorations in Group Work,* Boston: Milford House, pp. 17-72, 1973.

Mayadas, N. S. and O'Brien, D., "The Use of Videotape in Group Psychotherapy," *Group Therapy and Psychodrama,* Vol. 26, No. 1-2, pp. 107-119.

Rubin, Judith A. Child Art Therapy: *Understanding and Helping Children Grow through Art,* New York: Van Nostrand Reinhold Co., 288 pp., 1978.

Sontag, Susan, *On Photography,* New York: Farrar, Straus and Giroux, 1977.

Stewart, Doug. "Photo Therapy: Theory and Practice," *Art Psychotherapy,* Vol. 6, pp. 41-46, Pergamon Press, 1979.

Stoller, F. H. "Group Psychotherapy on T.V.: An Innovation with Hospitalized Patients," *American Psychologist,* Vol. 22, p. 158, 1967.

Stoller, F. H. "Videotape Feedback in the Group Setting," *Journal of Nervous and Mental Disease,* pp. 457-466, 1969.

Activities and Hispanic Groups: Issues and Suggestions

Melvin Delgado

ABSTRACT. The importance of using activities with Hispanic groups cannot be underestimated. However, activities must be based upon a sound understanding of cultural values and their influence on Hispanic attitudes and behaviors. This article will examine the role of activities in the treatment of Hispanic adults. In addition to reviewing the literature on use of activities with Hispanic groups, attention will be given to factors that facilitate the use of activities with Hispanics, and the relationship of goals, activities and role of group leader throughout the group developmental cycle.

INTRODUCTION

The importance of using activities with Hispanic groups cannot be underestimated. The limited use of group treatment for Hispanics may be attributed to the interplay of a variety of factors: (1) organizational barriers (type of setting, quality of the relationship between the setting and community, lack of bilingual staff, nature of group recruitment); (2) group process related issues (group expectations of what constitutes treatment, scheduling logistics, use of Spanish, group themes); (3) acculturation and value orientation of group members; and (4) group leadership limitations (differing expectations of the role of leader).

This article will examine the role of activities in the treatment of Hispanic adults. In addition to reviewing the literature on use of activities with Hispanic groups, attention will be given to factors that facilitate the use of activities with Hispanics, and the use of culturally sensitive activities throughout the various stages of group development.

Melvin Delgado is an Associate Professor at Boston University School of Social Work, 264 Bay State Rd., Boston, Mass. 02215. The author wishes to express his gratitude to Professors Louise Frey and Jim Garland, Boston University School of Social Work, for their contributions in helping to develop a conceptual foundation for this article.

85

FACTORS FACILITATING THE USE
OF ACTIVITIES WITH HISPANICS

The difficulties in recruiting and keeping Hispanics in treatment groups have been well documented in the literature (Herrera and Sanchez, 1976; Mizio, 1979; Smith and Miller, 1979). Nevertheless, group treatment has been successfully applied to a variety of Hispanic groups with differences in gender, age, presenting symptoms, and country of origin.

In reviewing the key themes raised in the literature on Hispanic groups, two in particular take on added significance for the use of activities. If Hispanic groups are to achieve therapeutic change, it is necessary for group leaders to (1) take an action-oriented approach that stresses issues group members are *currently* experiencing (Boulette, 1975:404), and (2) construct a supportive, non-competitive environment that stresses cooperation rather than competition.

The preference for an action-oriented focus can derive from any one or combination of the following aspects: (1) environmental demands (poverty, unresponsive social institutions, crisis); (2) locus of control may be perceived to exist outside of the individual (environment may be perceived to be uncontrollable, unpredictable, and hostile); and (3) cultural value orientation focuses on concrete solutions to present problems (Kluckhorn and Strodtbeck, 1961).

Delgado (1980:77), in applying the Kluckhorn and Strodtbeck Value Orientation Scale to Hispanic groups, notes the following in examining the importance of activity and time orientations on group functioning:

> Insight into personal problems should not constitute a significant role in (Hispanic) group treatment. Consequently, a group leader must refrain from fostering this attitude. Instead a value orientation stressing action requires development of concrete solutions. Group goals should be short- rather than long-term and easily measurable by the group. . . . A present time orientation stresses current problems and solutions. A group leader, in turn, must refrain from focusing on the past or future. His/her direction should be present-time oriented, helping the group to find solutions that, keeping in tune with a doing orientation, can be implemented immediately and are easily

measurable—in other words, action leading to behavior rather than attitude change.

According to Delgado, there is a highly significant relationship between activity and present-time value orientations.

In examining the group literature, it becomes apparent that certain themes are highly popular with Hispanic groups, along with the use of problem-solving techniques. Group themes generally fall into two categories: interpersonal or environmental. Interpersonal related themes usually focus on loneliness, unrealistic role expectations of themselves and others, somatic illness, depression and fatalism (Hynes and Werbin, 1977; Kraidman, 1980; Normand, Iglesias and Payn, 1977). Environmental related themes invariably focus on issues of discrimination, use of human resources, and hardships such as poor housing, personal and family safety, and lack of money (Brown and Arevalo, 1979; Menikoff, 1979; Werbin and Hynes, 1975; Cooper and Cento, 1977).

Reliance on problem-solving techniques with Hispanics serve to highlight several important interpersonal and environmental themes: (1) perceptions of the presenting problem(s) as being influenced by a variety of factors (group members will view situations/issues from various perspectives in order to find acceptable solutions); (2) effective communication skills are very important in preventing and solving problems (ability to communicate and actively listen); (3) understanding of decision-making processes (awareness of how and why human beings make decisions about themselves and others); (4) acknowledgement of the importance of support groups in the lives of individuals (natural groups such as a family or friends, or other types of groups); (5) the necessity for developing a plan of action to solve problems (problems require careful analysis and a deliberate attempt to seek solutions—in essence, problems do not magically disappear); and (6) the placing of the locus of control within the individual (a person with problems does have control over his/her environment in most instances).

Lastly, the necessity for providing a supportive environment based upon cooperation is crucial in order to address the themes covered above and in using problem-solving techniques. Qualities of independence and self-reliance are very often stressed within the American society. However, within the Hispanic culture, the opposite values of interdependence and cooperation are stressed (Arenas, 1978; Condon, Peters and Sueiro-Ross, 1979: 69-72,

110-111). Hispanics generally shy away from situations that result in "winners" and "losers." "Saving face" is of critical importance within the culture and competitive situations increase the likelihood of someone being embarrassed by losing. Consequently, activities that involve the entire group in a non-competitive environment will be well received.

GROUP ACTIVITIES AND GROUP DEVELOPMENTAL STAGES

Activities with groups can take on a variety of manifestations depending upon the needs of the members, the nature of the setting, and the skills and orientation of the group leader (Vinter, 1974: 233-234). Activities for Hispanic groups should attempt to achieve enhancement of individual well-being and facilitate the exercise of control over the environment (Alissi, 1980: 364-365). In similar fashion to other groups, activities must:

> . . . contain the possibility of successful accomplishment. It must be safe and interesting, as well as appropriate in terms of age, sex, cultural background, intellectual endowment, etc. It must be appropriate for the size of the group, size of the room, physical setting . . . and encompassable without alienating other groups meeting in the next room, the neighbors, or the community. (Middleman, 1968: 108)

In essence, in developing activities for use with Hispanic groups, many of the universal aspects are prevalent, along with unique cultural aspects.

Although the use of activities should be a central focus of the group, this is not to say that Hispanics cannot benefit from discussions pertaining to emotional difficulties (Cooper and Cento, 1977). However, activities should be the primary mechanisms from which to focus these discussions.

A wide range of activities has been utilized with Hispanic groups (e.g., physical exercises, field trips, advocacy projects, community recreation events), and these have proved very successful in attracting and maintaining Hispanics in groups. These group activities have attempted to meet instrumental (attainment of material goods and concrete services), emotional (support, counseling, etc.), and informational needs (childrearing, human services, individual rights, etc.).

For the purposes of analyzing the use of activities throughout the group development stages, Garland, Jones and Kolodny's conceptualization of group development will be utilized: (1) pre-affiliation; (2) power and control; (3) intimacy; (4) differentiation; and (5) separation (1973: 17-71). Each of these stages, in turn, will be examined from four perspectives: (1) factors that will influence the planning of activities; (2) goals; (3) examples of activities that are sensitive to cultural values; and (4) the role of group leader.

Pre-Affiliation Stages

Factors to consider. The recruitment and beginning phases of the group are crucial in dictating the nature and function of the group. Various factors must be considered regardless of the characteristics and needs of group members. First, the values of honor, dignity, and respect are of particular importance to Hispanics. Related characteristics, e.g., sense of equality, respect for differences, and regard for one's reputation, are closely associated with honor and dignity. As Leavitt (1974: 46) has indicated:

> The essence of the individual, his soul, is expressed by the value of dignity, which is guarded from insult and invasion by respecto (respect), a pattern of cercmonial politeness constantly observed by all but the closest relatives and friends.

Dignity, in turn, is also associated with confianza (confidence). Confianza expresses pure friendship, based on mutual understanding and appreciation, without obligations of kinship (Leavitt, 1974). Consequently, dignity and confidence serve to regulate behavior between family members, friends, neighbors, and strangers. These cultural values will be manifested in a group environment through an unwillingness to admit to personal problems, courteous behavior, and minimal sharing.

A second factor that must be considered during this stage of group development is closely related to the above values. The tendency to stress interdependence and cooperation will influence greatly the type of activities that should be developed. Effort must be made to produce a non-competitive environment; and the activities should not be excessively demanding or have a low probability of success. It is only after a series of activities (low on demand and high on success) have been accomplished that the group should attempt more complex and demanding assignments. In essence, success, par-

ticularly during the initial stages of group development, is of para-
mount importance.

Goals, activities and role of group leader. The goals, activities
and role of group leader will vary depending upon the nature of the
group and setting. However, as noted in Table I, a core can be identified that is applicable to Hispanic groups.

The group leader must endeavor to structure activities that are
culturally sensitive. The presence of food for the members is an important aspect in fostering a warm and accepting environment. Further, the use of exercises that attempt to enlist historical
backgrounds will serve to highlight members' similarities and differences. The pre-affiliation stage should be low key and allow
members sufficient flexibility to participate at their own pace. In
developing exercises, note must be made that all members may *not*
be able to read and write in either Spanish or English; consequently,
exercises should not be based upon written responses on the part of
the members.

Power and Control Stage

Factors to consider. Issues of power and control represent important aspects in daily life. In examining these two aspects from a
cultural perspective, important issues emerge. The traditional
Hispanic family is patriarchal, with the male head of household fulfilling a strong authoritarian role and the female a passive-
submissive role. Authority figures have traditionally not been ques-
tioned within Hispanic families. Taking this issue one step further,
poor Hispanics invariably are at the mercy of authorities, i.e.,
police, court officials, teachers, etc. Consequently, the authority
represented in the form of group leader may be viewed as absolute.

The authority of the group leader will eventually be challenged by
group members. However, the length of time that must transpire,
and the manner in which this will be manifested, will highlight
Hispanic cultural values. This stage in group development will
probably last much longer than otherwise experienced with other
racial and cultural groups; also, group members may expect the
group leader to act in similar fashion to other authority figures they
have encountered—"whatever you say is fine with us."

Goals, activities and role of group leader. In examining Table II,
cultural manifestations become apparent in the foods selected and
prepared by group members and the rotating of meeting sites among

TABLE I
Pre-Affiliation Stage of Group Development

GOALS	TYPE OF ACTIVITY	ROLE OF GROUP LEADER
1. Conducive environment	Group decides what they feel is important to achieve a conducive setting.	Facilitate the identification of factors; acquire room, food, etc.
2. Sharing of backgrounds	Brief historical review exercise (members introduce) each other and share what they learned about group members.	Help structure the exercise and share along with the group.
3. Identification of member expectations	Members list three important goals.	Help process the groups goals.
4. Contract	Group members will list concrete things they hope to achieve.	Provide leadership and guidance.

TABLE II
Power and Control Stage of Group Development

GOALS	TYPE OF ACTIVITY	ROLE OF GROUP LEADER
1. Development of a group sense of power and control over the course of events.	Group decides the type of food and setting rotation; develops a schedule.	Facilitate group decisions; provide transportation, etc.
2. Development of an understanding of decisionmaking.	Group develops a list of rules.	Highlight group decisionmaking process; restate group decisions.
3. Group development and selection of activities.	Group develops a list of activities and expectations.	Provide input and guidance; present ideas of types of activities.

group members. The latter activity allows each member to act as host and facilitates a sharing process.

The group leader, being cognizant of the importance of authority within the culture, should facilitate the group decision-making process. However, the leader should endeavor to participate in the process as much as possible. When he/she does not, mention should be made that it is not because the group leader does not care about the group, but the decision is really a group responsibility. It is important to remember that lack of involvement in the decision-making process can be interpreted by the group as a sign of not caring.

Failure of the group leader to be able to differentiate this important aspect may result in the group disbanding!

One activity that the author has found particularly useful with Hispanic groups has been to have members describe the three most important sources of supports in their lives. Invariably, depending upon individual circumstances, members list a variety of helpers: (1) family; (2) religious figures; (3) folk healers; and (4) community merchants and friends (Delgado and Humm-Delgado, 1982).

The group leader, in turn, helps the group identify common sources of support and highlights how these sources compare or differ with other racial and ethnic groups. By examining Hispanic natural support systems within the broader context of American society, members can appreciate their uniqueness. Reliance on folk healers, it must be noted, will rarely be shared in a public meeting unless there is a feeling of trust. Consequently, this factor may serve as an excellent indicator of group cohesion and trust.

Intimacy Stage

Factors to consider. This stage of group development is best characterized by "intensification of personal involvement, more willingness to bring into the open feelings regarding club members and worker striving for satisfaction of dependency needs. . . There is a growing awareness and mutual recognition of the significance of the group experience in terms of personality growth and change" (Garland, Jones and Kolodny, 1976: 47).

This stage may witness Hispanic group members stating that they "feel they are among family." The concept of family when placed within a cultural context will connote an important sense of belonging. It must be remembered that the definition of a family within the Hispanic culture goes beyond that of the nuclear family. The concept of compadrazo is an important link in the extended family network which unites distant relatives, friends, and neighbors in mutually supportive roles. Thus, it is very possible for several group members to become closely attached, or mention in the group that they feel as if they were among family.

Goals, activities and role of group leader. As indicated in Table III, this stage in group development intensifies group relations, encourages activities that are more complex, and involves the group leader in the sharing process.

The group leader's primary role will be to facilitate group pro-

TABLE III

Intimacy Stage of Group Development

GOALS	TYPE OF ACTIVITY	ROLE OF GROUP LEADER
1. Intensification of member involvement.	Group will plan activities outside of regular meetings- projects should involve several members.	Encourage outside meeting; provide technical support where needed.
2. Projects increase in complexity.	Activities invariably involve members in carrying out com- plimentary tasks.	Facilitate the carrying out of tasks; help pro- cess issues.
3. Increase sharing of personal issues.	Members are encouraged to share an issue/problem they would like to have the group resolve.	Facilitate and share when appro- priate.

jects by providing technical assistance (making phone calls, etc.), facilitating group sharing, and participating in the sharing when appropriate. Activities may range in scope and intensity. One activity that has proved particularly successful with Hispanic groups has been the planning of a field trip to another city. Invariably these types of activities involve family members and friends, and serve to introduce the group leader to family members.

Differentiation Stage

Factors to consider. This stage of group development will manifest itself in group members' accepting one another as individuals and seeing "this group experience as a unique experience from which each can find an acceptable intrapsychic equilibrium" (Garland, Jones and Kolodny, 1976: 52). This stage should encourage the identification of commonalities and differences among group members. Differences, in turn, must be accepted by members. Effort must be made to generalize these discoveries to the "outside world." It should be noted that the value of interdependence that is often associated with this stage of development is also a cultural value!

Goals, activities and role of group leader. As noted in Table IV, the group leader plays a minimal role in this stage of development other than facilitating the group process. Activities, in turn, may be minimal or non-existent. The group may be satisfied to meet and discuss personal issues without having to rely on activities.

Separation Stage

Factors to consider. This final stage in group development will often prove to be the most painful for Hispanic groups. The group member reactions listed by Garland, Jones and Kolodny (1973: 58-62), i.e., denial, regression, etc., will be present in Hispanic groups. In addition, separation will rekindle for some feelings associated with leaving their country of origin. The group leader must be prepared to continue his/her relationship with individual members after the group has terminated—"will you visit me and my family?"

This latter factor is particularly associated with Hispanics. The group leader, depending upon the intensity of the relationship with the group, will be asked to participate in family affairs and celebrations. In essence, the leader should not necessarily view these invitations as a failure in properly terminating with the group. Similar occurrences are prevalent in one-to-one relationships; in fact, he/she may be asked to be a godparent to a child.

Goals, activities and role of group leader. In similar fashion to the differentiation stage of group development, separation will not require extensive use of activities with possibly one exception—a celebration to mark the successful ending of the group. Table V highlights components of this stage.

TABLE IV
Differentiation Stage of Group Development

GOALS	TYPE OF ACTIVITY	ROLE OF GROUP LEADER
1. Explore group member differences/similarities.	Group members share some of the more striking similarities/differences.	Facilitate and share.
2. Compare group experiences with others.	Same as above.	Same as above.

TABLE V
Separation Stage of Group Development

GOALS	TYPE OF ACTIVITY	ROLE OF GROUP LEADER
1. Review group progress and experiences.	Every group member may be expected to share.	Facilitate and share.
2. Feelings concerning termination should be raised.	Same as above.	Same as above.
3. Celebration.	Plan and carry out.	Facilitate.

The planning of a formal celebration to mark the termination of the group is very often an excellent activity to bring together group members and their families. Also, if this has not occurred during other stages of group development, it will be important for the group member's family to meet the group leader.

CONCLUSION

This article has examined the literature on Hispanic groups and highlighted factors that are important in setting the foundation for use of activities. In addition, goals, activities and role of group leader have been described according to five stages of group development.

The use of a group modality to meet the needs of Hispanics has not been sufficiently utilized in human service settings. However, this modality has great potential for assisting Hispanics. The use of activities in the planning and development of Hispanic groups is an excellent means of recruiting and maintaining Hispanics in groups. These activities, however, must be based on a sound understanding of cultural values; failure to take culture into consideration will result in failure for the group leader!

REFERENCES

Alissi, A.S. Comparative group methods. In A.S. Alissi, Ed., *Perspectives on social group work practice: A book of readings.* New York: The Free Press, 1980.

Arenas, S. Bilingual/bicultural programs for preschool children. *Children Today,* 1978, July-August, 2-6.

Boulette, T.R. Group therapy for low income Mexican Americans. *Social Work,* 1975, *20,* 403-406.

Brown, J.A. & Arevalo, R. Chicanos and social group work models: Some Implications for group work practice. *Social Work with Groups,* 1979, *2,* 331-342.

Condon, E.C., Peters, J. & Sueiro-Ross, C. *Special education and the Hispanic child: Cultural dimensions.* Philadelphia: Teacher Corps Mid-Atlantic Network, Temple University, 1979.

Delgado, M. Hispanic cultural values: Implications for groups. *Small Group Behavior,* 1981, *12,* 69-80.

Delgado, M. & Humm-Delgado, D. Natural support systems: Source of strength in Hispanic communities. *Social Work,* 1982, *27.*

Garland, J., Jones, H.E. & Kolodny, R.L. A model for stages of development in social work groups. In S. Bernstein, Ed. Explorations in group work. Boston: Charles River Press, 1973.

Herrera, A.E. & Sanchez, V.C. Behaviorally oriented group therapy: A successful application in the treatment of low income Spanish-speaking clients. In M. Miranda, Ed., *Psychotherapy for the Spanish-speaking.* Los Angeles: Spanish-Speaking Mental Health Research Center, 1976.

Hynes, K. & Werbin, J. Group psychotherapy for Spanish-speaking women. *Psychiatric Annals,* 1977, *7,* 52-63.

Kluckhohn, F.R. & Strodtbeck, F.L. Variations in value orientations. Evanston, Ill: Row, Peterson, 1961.

Kraidman, M. Group therapy with Spanish-speaking clinic patients to enhance ego functioning. *Group*, 1980, *4*, 59-64.

Leavitt, R.R. *The Puerto Rican: Culture change and language deviance.* Tucson, Ariz.: Viking Fund Publishions in Anthropology, 1974.

Maes, W. & Rivaldi, J.R. Counseling the Chicano child. *Elementary School Guidance and Counseling,* 1974, *8*, 279-284.

Martinez, C. Group process and the Chicano: Clinical issues. *International Journal of Group Psychotherapy,* 1977, *27*, 225-231.

Menikoff, A. Long-term group psychotherapy for Puerto Rican Women: Ethnicity as a clinical support. *Group,* 1979, *3*, 172-180.

Middleman, R.R. *The non-verbal method in working with groups.* New York: Association Press, 1968.

Mizio, E. *Puerto Rican task force report.* New York: Family Service Association of America, 1979.

Normand, W.C., Iglesias, J. & Payn, S. Brief group therapy to facilitate utilization of mental health services by Spanish-speaking patients. *American Journal of Orthopsychiatry,* 1974, *44*, 37-42.

Smith, D. & Miller, R. Personal growth groups: A comparison of the experiences of Anglo and Mexicans. *Small Group Behavior,* 1979, *10*, 263-270.

Unger, D.G. & Powell, D.R. Supporting families under stress: The role of social networks. *Family Relations,* 1980, *29*, 566-574.

Vinter, R.D. Program activities: An analysis of their effects on participant behavior. In P. Glasser, R. Sarri & R. Vinter, Eds., *Individual change through small groups.* New York: The Free Press, 1974.

Werbin, J. & Hynes, K. Transference and culture in a Latino group. *International Journal of Group Psychotherapy,* 1975, *25*, 396-401.

BOOK REVIEWS

SELF-HELP GROUPS FOR COPING WITH CRISIS. Morton A. Lieberman, Leonard D. Borman, and Associates. *San Francisco: Jossey-Bass Publishers, 1979, 462 pages.*

This volume addresses a relatively neglected topic that is of interest to many group work practitioners, namely, self-help groups. The authors draw upon a number of writers, including graduate students from the University of Chicago, to prepare seventeen chapters, plus an overview and a conclusion section. The volume focuses upon four major areas: (1) how self-help groups are started and structured, (2) who participates in self-help groups, (3) how self-help groups work, and (4) evaluating the impact of self-help groups. In essence, the authors limit their investigation to historical, ethnographic, and survey studies about a small cluster of self-help organizations. These include Alcoholics Anonymous, Synanon, Mended Hearts, Compassionate Friends, Naim (a self-help group for the widowed), SAGE (a self-help group for the elderly), and consciousness-raising groups for women.

In commenting upon the growth and development of self-help groups, the authors emphasize how helping professionals typically have founded, supported, and complemented the activities of such entities. This perspective differs from a commonly accepted notion, to wit, that self-help organizations tend to compete with, or supplant, the efforts of helping professionals. They note that the latter have assisted self-help groups by progressing beyond the conventional theories of the day, defining pertinent afflictions in a broader or more innovative fashion, expanding the skills and techniques of self-help organizations, focusing on problem stages or conditions that usually are neglected by other observers, and showing a strong concern for seriously neglected populations. Likewise, helping professionals have stimulated the growth of self-help groups by altering professional roles in a constructive manner, creating new auspices

97

for self-help groups, developing innovative ways of recruiting members, and reducing service fees.

Many of the chapters in the volume are case studies of selected self-help groups. Though the authors strive to collate and synthesize convergent trends from these chapters, their empirical generalizations must be viewed with caution in view of sampling and methodological limitations. Indeed, many of the deficiencies of field research concerning self-help groups are recognized by the authors and are discussed in the last four chapters of the book. For the most part, however, the interested reader would learn a great deal more about evaluating self-help groups by referring to standard texts concerning evaluation research. The limited research which appears in the volume tends to be somewhat equivocal in nature. Though certain of the self-help groups seemed to yield measureable benefits for their members, others did not. Somewhat conservatively, the authors conclude, at least, that such groups seem to produce very few negative consequences for their members.

Those sections of the volume which examine change processes within small groups are likely to be of greatest interest to group work practitioners. In Chapter 10 ("Analyzing Change Mechanisms of Groups"), Lieberman merely rank orders questionnaire items which presumably denote group members' perceptions about the experiences and events that they found helpful in self-help groups. Leon Levy, in Chapter 11 ("Processes and Activities in Groups") cites a number of basic processes that characterize self-help groups. Thus, for example, they presumably remove members' mystification about their experiences, increase expectancies for change, provide rationales for problems and for the group's way of dealing with them, offer normative or instrumental information and advice, and expand alternative perceptions about problems and ways of resolving them. Likewise, they enhance members' discriminative abilities regarding the stimulus and event contingencies in their lives, provide support for attitudinal changes toward oneself, one's own behavior, and society, reduce members' uncertainty and sense of isolation about their problems, enhance processes of social comparison and consensual validation, and provide alternative social structures within which members can develop new personal identities and new behavioral norms.

Perhaps the most innovative and useful contributions in the volume pertain to the authors' efforts to explicate the role of "ideologies" in enhancing the work of self-help groups. In Chapter

12 ("Role of Ideologies in Peer Psychotherapy Groups"), for instance, Paul Antze highlights how this much neglected desideratum exerts an impact upon the development and therapeutic effectiveness of groups sponsored by Alcoholics Anonymous, Recovery Incorporated, and Synanon. In Chapter 13 ("Emergence of Ideology in a Bereaved Parent Group"), Barry Sherman further examines the linkage between ideology and therapeutic change. Though the volume is not likely to be of interest to most group work practitioners, it undoubtedly should be brought to the attention of professionals who are concerned specifically about self-help groups. Practice principles appear rarely within the book. But, nonetheless, the volume draws together various findings about self-help groups that appear even more rarely, if it all, in other compendiums concerning this general topic.

Ronald A. Feldman
Professor of Social Work
Washington University, St. Louis

IDENTIFYING, MEASURING AND TEACHING HELPING SKILLS. Lawrence Shulman. *New York: Council on Social Work Education, 1981; Ottawa, Ontario: Canadian Association of Schools of Social Work, 1981, 146 pp.*

"This book attempts to address the need in social work education to identify the skills required for effective practice, to develop instruments to measure these skills, and to design an approach to teach them effectively." Unfortunately the objectives of this book were not achieved.

The book consists of four chapters; one chapter addresses the identification of helping skills, two chapters address the measurement of helping skills and the final chapter addresses the teaching of helping skills. The first chapter is the cornerstone of Shulman's efforts. In this chapter Shulman argues for greater specificity in the identification of helper treatment skills. He contends that what is often missing in studies of helper client contacts are insights into the actual "interactions" that took place during treatment. He encourages greater elaboration in the identification of helping behaviors and suggests examining the client worker *interaction* in relation to treatment outcomes, rather than focusing solely on outcome. He draws from the work of William Schwartz and uses Schwartz's mediational model of helping as both his working and conceptual foundation. The author outlines the phases of worker client interactions as envisioned by Schwartz and identifies twenty-seven worker activities which he views as beneficial to the helping process, e.g. clarifying purpose, displaying feelings openly.

In the second chapter Shulman outlines his attempts to gather data on client-worker interactions. He constructs a questionnaire, The Social Worker Behavior Questionnaire, by converting the worker activities (helping skills) into questions. For example, helping skill #1 Clarifying Purpose was converted to the statement, "In our first meeting my worker explained the kinds of concerns we might be discussing." Clients were asked to report the extent to which their workers engaged in each of the 27 helping skills: (1) often, (2) fairly often, (3) seldom, (4) never, or (5) no answer. A great portion of this chapter is spent in review of problems incurred in construction of the research instrument, The Social Worker Behavior Questionnaire. However, Shulman is scant in his descriptions of clients and practitioners, nor does he adequately describe his research methodology. He does, however, identify the numerous limitations of the study and informs the reader of the studies' lack of experimental design and rigor. Results of the study were modest. Of those twenty-seven helping skills identified, "skilled" and "unskilled" workers were found to differ significantly on only two of these. Similarly with respect to the worker's educational level, (AB, BS, MSW) clients reported receiving no consistent or discriminating differences in the perceived helping skills of these practitioners. That is, each of these educational groups scored higher on some helping skills than did the other two groups.

In the third chapter Shulman outlines his development of an observational system of measuring worker client interactions, the Social Work Interaction Analysis Category. This instrument is very similar to the Social Work Behavioral Questionnaire. However, the SWINC contains thirteen rather than twenty-seven interaction categories. He informs us that such an observation system provides a means for making systematic recordings of interactions between workers and clients. Shulman requires individual raters to classify videoed interactions between workers and clients using the SWINC as a means of measurement. This effort resulted in a quantitative description of the worker client interactions as they were classified according to the thirteen categories. He then offers a discussion of the interactions between the thirteen categories, which consist of an inspection of how certain categories followed one another, e.g., "worker encourages elaboration of theme of concern" was often followed by "worker listens while the client talks." However, Shulman does not discuss the utility of such quantitative data as it affects either client satisfaction or treatment outcomes. For example, it would be useful to know if successful workers engage in some categories longer or more frequently than unsuccessful workers and/or does the ratio of time spent in certain categories rather than in others result in improved service to clients.

The final chapter addresses the issue of teaching helping skills. The author offers some good ideas for teaching in general, but none appeared to be derived from the empirically focused efforts outlined in chapters two and three of the book. Instead, based on his personal experiences, the author makes a series of analogies between the skills employed in classroom teaching and those skills needed for practice with clients. It is curious that the author conducted empirical studies to measure helping skills and then chose not to utilize knowledge derived from that research in the teaching of such skills. In view of his research findings, this fourth chapter on teaching helping skills is premature and might well have been deferred until those practitioner skills or activities which are associated with client improvement, and/or satisfaction have been more adequately identified and measured.

Larry E. Davis
Professor
George Warren Brown School of Social Work
Washington University
St. Louis

ROLE PLAYING: A PRACTICAL MANUAL FOR GROUP
FACILITATORS. Malcolm Shaw, Raymond Corsin, Robert Blake,
Jane S. Mouton. *San Diego: University Associates, Inc. 1980,
202 pages.*

"Role Play" is not a new group technique. Its use in teaching and
training has been frequently referred to in the literature of group
work. It has been used to rehearse behavior, to provide situations
for discussion, and to sensitize group participants to the attitudes
and behaviors inherent in particular roles. As the use of role play
has increased, however, there has been a growing need to crystalize
the guidelines which can make for an efficient, effective use of the
technique. This approach enables role play to become more than
something to do to fill time.

Role Playing: A Practical Manual for Group Facilitators meets
many of those needs experienced by practitioners and its entrance
into the literature on Role Playing is most welcome.

The authors make it very clear, both in the book's title and in its
content, that the book is written for group facilitators and, although
some content addresses teachers and trainers, it is geared primarily
to companies, organizations and management centers (as opposed to
social service agencies or schools, for example). Lest this be viewed
as a reason not to use the book, it should be mentioned that the
material presented can be expanded (or contracted) by the reader to
use in many varied situations. Chapter 8 on Training and Chapter 10
on Modifying Behavior are examples of material that will stretch to
accommodate the needs of the user—needs that are reflected in other
disciplines and other professions.

The book is laid out in three separate sections and has an excellent
annotated bibliography and three appendices which give case
material and provide observers guides and role-players rating
sheets.

The first section deals with the background of Role Playing.
Although this section is brief considering the wealth of material that
could have been covered, it does give a solid foundation, both
theoretical and practical, on which the following sections are based.

The second section deals with techniques of Role Playing. It is
here where one finds the essence of the authors formulations. The
definitions and descriptions of Structured and Unstructured Role
Playing are crisp and clear. Missing from this section is consideration of what might be called "semi-structured" role playing, which

builds more on the collaboration of facilitators and group than the aforementioned designs which place responsibilities or either the facilitator or group members.

The authors discuss four components of role playing: climate setting, action, feedback and generalizing. And although these sections are, again, concise and useful, recognition and discussion of the environment in which the role play takes place (not the environment of the group) would have strengthened the validity of the role play action. The Chapter on specific techniques provides solid material for those who want to add to their basic role playing skills. A caveat might be in order for the technique of doubling—be clear as to who is being doubled—the *role* or the *person* playing the role. The proscribed nature of the played role may be substantially different from the person playing the role both in attitude and behavior. Some guidelines on debriefing might have proved helpful since an extended role play can become very intense and self-absorbing even in a non-clinical setting.

The third section deals with the application of Role Playing and examines Informing, Training, Evaluating and Modifying Behavior and it is in this section that one finds clues to a broader use of the role playing techniques.

For the worker (or facilitator) who has been engaged in role playing, this book will be a good resource. For that person unfamiliar or relatively new to role playing it will provide much helpful information.

Edmond T. Jenkins
Associate Professor of Social Work
School of Applied Social Sciences
Case Western Reserve University

DYNAMICS OF GROUP DECISION. Hermann Brandstatter, James Davis, and Heinz Schuler. *Beverly Hills: Sage Publications, 1978, 276 pages.*

This book is a collection of papers presented at a symposium sponsored by the European Association of Experimental Social Psychology and its American counterpart, the Society of Experimental Social Psychologists. The symposium was held in Ottobeuron Germany in 1978. The papers are reports of specific European and British research projects which have examined some aspect of group decision making. The exception to this is the inclusion of work by James Davis and his students or former students at the University of Illinois.

This volume illustrates the diversity in focus of attention (i.e., subject matter), methodological approaches and theoretical assumptions of contemporary small group research. It could hardly do otherwise. Papers included in the volume cover rather discrete, ethnocentric and narrow perspectives. It is regrettable that papers given at an international symposium give little evidence that the authors are aware of previous or current research going on in the other countries represented. The citations used provide an obvious example of this. Psychology is the primary discipline represented in these papers and the primary "focus" of attention. One might expect that this limitation would bring some unity. It does not.

The pages are organized into three categories and are intended to illustrate research in that area: (1) "Cooperative interaction: cognitive aspects"; what is typically called "group performance" in American small group literature; (2) "Cooperative interations: social emotive aspects"; what is typically called "group process" in social work literature and (3) "Mixed-motive interaction"; "bargaining," "negotiation" and/or "conflict resolution" in American small group literature. The four "group performance" papers are concerned with jury decisions, risk taking in group decisions, and cognitive development as a result of social interaction. The focus of attention of the research reports illustrating "group process" include two papers on the effect of friendliness, one paper on vicarious social reinforcement, and one paper on the influence of experts in group decision making. Mixed motive interaction articles include two research reports on bargaining and negotiation and one on reward allocation and intermember relations. Many of the findings of these studies are highly abstract and/or so tied to experimental conditions that they would be difficult to test in social work practice settings.

The very problems inherent in this work, demonstrate why such a book is valuable. American research and literature on the small group is quite provincial with research on decision making seemingly even more so. The book gives one a perspective and a glimpse of the differential methodology and content focus utilized in Great Britain and Western Europe.

Charles D. Cowger
Associate Professor
School of Social Work
University of Illinois, Urbana-Champaign

Call for Abstracts and Papers

Abstracts of papers or brief descriptions of presentations (workshops, media presentations, simulations, etc.) are to be submitted no later than **March 30, 1983.** They should be 250-500 words long and include a statement about main topic and basic premises. Where appropriate, reference should be made to empirical support for premises. Please indicate: (1) what sort of audience participation is intended; (2) length of time desired (min./max.); and (3) whether you are directing your presentation at a particular audience (e.g., new practitioners, teachers of groupwork, etc.)

Notification of Abstract acceptance will be made by **April 30, 1983.** Three copies of completed papers (approximate length of 15 pages) or details of other types of presentations are due on **June 30, 1983.** Acceptance of the abstract guarantees a place on the final program, providing the completed paper or details of other type of presentation is consistent with the approved abstract.

Send abstracts and papers to: Harvey Bertcher, Conference Chairperson, 4060 B Frieze Building, School of Social Work, The University of Michigan, Ann Arbor, Michigan 48109. (313) 763-6571.

For further information contact the University of Michigan Department of Conferences, 412 Maynard Street, Ann Arbor, Michigan 48109. (313) 764-5304.

The Advancement of Social Work with Groups

Fifth Annual Symposium
October 20-22, 1983

The Feedback Loop: Practice to Theory To Practice

Westin Hotel, Renaissance Center
Detroit, Michigan

The Advancement of Social Work with Groups

Fifth Annual Symposium
October 20-22, 1983

The Feedback Loop: Practice to Theory to Practice

Westin Hotel, Renaissance Center, Detroit, Michigan

A unique feature of the 1983 Symposium will be a number of sessions related to solving particular practice problems. A series of meetings on each topic will be conducted using a format in which (1) an opening paper will be presented that identifies key issues and raises practice questions; (2) practice-oriented presentations will describe ways of dealing with the problem (workshop sessions may provide further opportunity for participants to engage with the problem and proposed strategies.); (3) theory and research-oriented papers will focus on conceptual issues related to the problem; and (4) a concluding session will identify progress made during the previous sessions and will point to further work that needs to be done.

We shall select the problem areas through categorizing the abstracts received for the Symposium. We consequently urge you to submit proposals related to practice problems and their solutions.

Examples of practice areas and related practice problems in which interest has been expressed include, but are not restricted to:

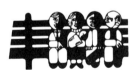

Developing new groupwork services (e.g., working with non-groupwork oriented administrators and staff; handling organizational resistance to group services.)

Unique problems of open-ended and/or changing membership groups

Groupwork in administrative practice (e.g., the mature staff group; strengthening teamwork in agency settings.)

Social groupwork and family issues

Problems of the unemployed

Empowerment through group participation (e.g., promoting member initiative)

Revitalizing field instruction

Minority status and social groupwork

Reducing violence with groupwork strategies

Groupwork for learning contexts

Gender issues and social groupwork (e.g., unique dilemmas for female leaders)

Papers that do not fit the above structure WILL ALSO BE INCLUDED in the program. The overall plan, in addition, includes plenary sessions on topics of concern to all, as well as sessions devoted to issues identified at the 1982 Symposium.

The FIFTH ANNUAL SYMPOSIUM is sponsored jointly by the following groups: Committee for the Advancement of Social Work with Groups, The Journal of Social Work with Groups, Haworth Press, Planning Committee consisting of representatives from agencies and social work programs (graduate and undergraduate) throughout Michigan and from Windsor, Ontario. In cooperation with the University of Michigan Extension Service.

CALL FOR PAPERS

Special Edition of *Social Work with Groups:* "Time-Limited Groups."

Under the Dual Guest Editorship of A.S. Alissi and Max Casper.

You are invited to submit manuscripts dealing with different aspects of social group work practice, theory and research on time-limited group experiences:

* The use of short-term frames in practice
* The single session group experience
* On-going group structures with changing memberships
* Differential use of skills, techniques and methods in long-term, short-term and single session groups

Manuscript is due by September 1, 1983.

Manuscripts may be submitted to the Guest Editors or to the Editors of *Social Work with Groups.* Please refer to Instructions for Authors.

Albert S. Alissi, University of Connecticut, School of Social Work, Greater Hartford Campus, West Hartford, Conn. 06117.

Max Casper, Syracuse University, School of Social Work, Brockway Hall, Syracuse, New York 13210.

ERRATUM

The following affiliation was omitted from publication for Elaine Bresler, CSW. It should have appeared with her article, "Filling an Empty Universe: Poetry Therapy with a Group of Emotionally Isolated Men," in *Social Work with Groups,* Volume 5, Number 3, Fall 1982.

Elaine Bresler, CSW, is employed as a therapist by Westchester Jewish Community Services, a family mental health clinic. She is also a Certified Poetry Therapist and a board member of the National Association of Poetry Therapy.

We apologize for this oversight.

The Editors

ERRATUM

Due to oversights in the production of *Social Work with Groups,* Volume 5, Number 2, the article "The Group: A Chance at Human Connection for the Mentally Impaired," by Judith A. Lee, was published with typographical errors appearing in the author's article abstract and in the quote by T. S. Eliot.

We would like to run those portions of the article correctly and as the author intended.

Our apologies to the author and the readers.

ABSTRACT. This article describes an effective summer day program for the mentally impaired elderly. It discusses and illustrates the helping principles applied in a life model and interactionally oriented group milieu approach. A sense of self is restored through doing talking, and sharing common feelings. The provision of a positive here and now experience which recognizes and bolsters strengths makes it more attractive to live more fully here and now. Even the most regressed patients improved in outlook and functioning as a result of the group experience.

> I grow old . . . I grow old . . .
> I shall wear white flannel trousers,
> and walk upon the beach
> I have heard the mermaids singing,
>   each to each.
> I do not think they will sing
>   to me.
>
> T.S. Eliot